Born in Calabria in 1960, Vincenzo Brancatisano is a freelance journalist with a degree in law. He is also the co-author of *Speciale Di Bella*, a magazine dedicated to Luigi Di Bella. He lives in Modena.

Di Bella

The Man, the Cure, a Hope for All

Vincenzo **Brancatisano**

Translated by **Vicki Satlow**

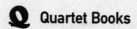 Quartet Books

First published in Great Britain by Quartet Books Limited in 1998
A member of the Namara Group
27 Goodge Street
London W1P 2LD

A catalogue record for this book is available from the British Library

ISBN   0 7043 8093 5

Printed and bound in Great Britain by Cox & Wyman, Reading, Berks

Contents

Acknowledgements

I would first like to acknowledge all those afflicted with a tumour. Their testimonies, far more extensive than those reported in these pages, have allowed me to clearly see the path that, to Professor Luigi Di Bella, has been clear for over twenty years.

I am profoundly thankful to Professor Di Bella for his great humanity.

I would also like to thank: Adolfo and Giuseppe Di Bella for their friendship. I am immensely grateful to the courageous staff of "Modena Amica". Massimiliano Ranellucci and Enza Poltronieri were among the first to believe in the news I brought to the paper. I admire Celestino Zanfi for not submitting to pressure. Thanks also to Franco Fondriest and Gabriella Cianconi of the "movimento consumatori", and thanks to Gianfranco and Laura for their encouragement. Thanks to my mother and father for believing in me, and to Stevie and Vicki for believing in this book. Thanks to Professor Piero Guerzoni for his understanding.

Above all, my love and gratitude go to Carla who bathed me in attention and affection when I should have been giving it to her.

Vincenzo Brancatisano

The Man

Humble Beginnings

Luigi Di Bella was born in 1912, in the tiny village of Linguaglossa in the province of Catania, Sicily. Today, its old, tumbledown stone houses seem picturesque, nestling in meadows at the foot of Mount Etna. Over eighty years ago, however, it was a poor region, whose inhabitants scraped a living by farming. The majority of the population lived in poverty, more or less, and the Di Bellas were no exception.

Although he has rarely had the opportunity to return to Linguaglossa, Luigi Di Bella harbours fond memories of its winding streets, the church bells in its little piazza, the dark thunderings of the nearby volcano and the sudden lightning flashes which lit up its distant crater and illuminated the night sky.

Until recently most of the people living in Linguaglossa today (including Di Bella's distant relatives) were completely ignorant of the fact that the legendary scientist is actually their village's most famous son. The owner of the local newsstand admits that, although everyone now talks of little else, no-one spoke of the professor at all until a few months ago. Now the villagers are even thinking of organising a festival in his honour.

Luigi's father, Giuseppe, abandoned his university studies when he fell in love with Carmella Turnaturi, and they decided to get married. By that time, he had enough skill in dealing with letters and accounts to be able to earn his living assisting the villagers as a kind of unofficial solicitor. He was a resourceful man, capable of turning his hand to most trades, and the older villagers can remember him filling in for the local artisans, though, he was often only paid with food for his services. Somehow he managed to support his growing family, though the Di Bellas lived in extreme poverty. Their only real resource was a small plot of land they owned on the slopes of Etna. In time, however, even that gradually dwindled away: some of it was sold off, and the rest was devoured by the encroaching dust and lava of the volcano.

When Di Bella was born, on 17 July 1912, his mother Carmella had already given birth to twelve other children, three of whom died as infants. Luigi was a shy and quiet boy, very close to his mother. With the help of his sister Anna, an elementary school teacher, he learned to read and write by the time he was four. Discovering books opened a new world to him, and reading became his passion. All else was forgotten when he had a book in his hand. At home, the family ate only one meal a day, and even then, Luigi kept a book in front of him.

All the children in the family were expected to do something to contribute to the family's finances. The professor recalls spending many days collecting hazelnuts: 'I would have liked to buy a loaf of bread, I was so hungry; but I knew how important it was to save money.' The frugal habits he learned as a child he has retained later in life.

In order to study, Luigi borrowed his brothers' and sisters' books, and read them at night. Since there was no money to spare for lamp oil, the boy was often seen pacing outside, reading by the light of the street lamps. He felt an attraction to medicine from a very early age and still recalls how, as a boy, he tried to cure his friends' ailments with concoctions of locally gathered herbs.

When he finished elementary school, it was presumed by his family that Luigi would leave school and begin to earn his living. But the boy refused to abandon his learning.

Fortunately, one of his teachers had noticed his exceptional abilities and arranged for him to continue studying. The local priest taught him Latin, which was then required for the high school entrance exam and, within weeks, Luigi had made outstanding progress, and was able to translate complex passages with relative ease. Di Bella now speaks at least five languages. His perseverance was rewarded at the end of his summer holidays, when he was accepted into

Messina's competitive Liceo Scientifico, a high school where the emphasis was on science.

Antonio De Carlo, an old school friend, remembers Di Bella well from his high school days and wrote him a letter when, in 1973, the international media reported on Di Bella's extraordinary results in leukaemia research: "We all knew you were destined to do something extraordinary" he wrote. "We used to ask each other, 'Whatever happened to Luigi Di Bella?' And someone joked that you had discovered a wonderful substance that turned a battlefield into a party, with enemy soldiers dancing instead of shooting."

Having finished high school, Luigi enrolled to study medicine at the University of Messina. He found lodgings with his brothers in a run-down, pre-fab building erected after the devastating 1908 earthquake. To pay his way, he took on odd jobs, working in a pharmacy for a brief period, a position which gave him ample opportunity to satisfy his curiosity about medicine and pharmaceuticals. His finances were also helped by the scholarship he won for four consecutive years, as the most promising student of the region. Despite his difficult financial situation, he sent this money to his family, and supported himself only from his work.

It was during his time at university that he met and fell in love with Francesca Costa, the local pharmacist's young daughter, who eventually became his wife. Luigi often visited the Costas' house late in the evening after he had finished his studies. The doctor jokes that, while he was captivated initially by her blue eyes and pretty face, he was really drawn to Francesca's good-natured personality and incredible tolerance. Painfully shy, Di Bella never imagined that such an attractive young woman could be interested in him. He was too timid to confess his feelings to anyone so, for many months, he would visit her house under various pretences so he could spend time with her. Francesca used to tell her sons many years later that she was moved by the intensity of her young suitor's feelings for her; she knew instinctively that she would spend the rest of her life with this young man.

Meanwhile, Di Bella transferred to the University of Bari in order to continue studying under his physiology professor, Pietro Tullio, a well-known authority in his field. In July of 1936 (having voluntarily added twelve optional exams to the mandatory courses of his major) he graduated with the highest grades and full honours from the Faculty of Medicine. He was just 24 years old. He found work immediately as Assistant Professor at the Institute of Human Physiology in the Univeristy of Parma, then in 1937 he became Assistant Professor of Human Physiology at the University of Modena.

In 1941, Di Bella's first child was born, a son named Giuseppe after his grandfather. But the family's joy was short-lived, for soon afterwards the professor was drafted into the war, and sent to Greece as the captain of a medical team and director of a field hospital. In a short time, news of his medical expertise spread, with even the German military requesting his services. A picture of his resourcefulness and of his qualities as a doctor emerges from his orders that the land surrounding the camp be dug up and planted to supplement the hospital's meagre rations. He also had goats and cattle brought in to provide milk for the sick. His devotion to his patients' well-being is one of Di Bella's primary characteristics. On one occasion during the war, he insisted on giving up his horse on a long march so that a patient could make the journey more comfortably. During this period, he worked incessantly, rarely sleeping more than four hours a night, still a habit of his today.

Unfortunately military service took its toll on Di Bella's health and in 1943 he was repatriated, having contracted a severe case of malaria. For the last years of the war, Di Bella returned to his position at the University of Modena, and continued to teach. To escape the bombings (his house was near the railway station, a prime target) he and his family were evacuated to the small community of Bastiglia, a few miles outside Modena. With his wife Francesca, the baby Guiseppe and his sisters-in-law Citta and Sara, he moved into a shared farmhouse belonging to the Plessi family. "There were fifteen of us in that house," recalls Pia Plessi, then thirteen years old. "There were two rooms, and only one was heated. The professor used to see patients from Bastiglia every morning. Many people came to be trated by him at our house; his treatment was always free of charge."

During this time, Di Bella had his own health problems to contend with: his malaria periodically plagued him with chills and high fevers. But he fought it with enormous vitality, refusing to allow the illness to curtail his activities. Regardless of both the bombs and his fever, he went to Modena daily on his bicycle to teach his classes at the university.

On the 30 December 1947, Luigi and Francesca's second son, Adolfo, was born. Shortly afterwards, an epidemic of pneumonia swept through Modena, to which the doctor discovered he had been exposed. Fearful of spreading the disease to his family, he sent them to Messina to stay with his in-laws. The Di Bellas remained there until 1953, the professor making regular trips to Sicily to visit them.

Upon moving back to Modena, the Di Bellas went on seeing the Plessi family occasionally, and the professor continued to treat patients from their village. Pia Plessi recalls that he once completely cured her sister of a serious thyroid complaint with a novel treatment based on brewer's yeast.

On another occasion, when an aunt was afflicted with terrible pains in her joints which confounded specialists, Di Bella accurately diagnosed her with a tumour of the spinal chord. The subsequent operation that he recommended arrested her condition, and she made a complete recovery. Her neighbours were amazed to see the old lady up and cycling around the countryside some months later – in fact, she lived to the ripe old age of 87.

Despite the enormous amount of time the professor has always dedicated to his studies and his patients, he was an active, and strict, father. Adolfo, his younger son, is now fifty, and married with two children (the boy is named after his grandfather Luigi). Adolfo has inherited his father's passion for music, and composes classical pieces in his spare time. Nowadays, most of his time is dedicated to organising his father's agenda. Every other Saturday, after finishing his work in a bank, Adolfo Di Bella goes directly to Modena's Via Marianini to clear his father's desk as well. The correspondence which the doctor receives each week threatens to take over the whole office. Adolfo tries his best to ease his father's workload, and to deal with the hundreds of patients requesting his help, but he has to make them understand that his father simply cannot take on any more patients.

The father–son relationship offers an insight into the personality of this very private man. 'He used to tell his friends about everything we did when we were children,' remembers Adolfo. 'Even the most silly things. It was really from other people that we came to understand how proud he was of us and our successes.'

As the boys matured, their father's affection deepened into a wider concern for their education and their futures. 'Even though his commitment to his work meant he was often away from home, he still managed to look after the family and participate actively in our upbringing,' says his son. 'Since he was always at the university working, he used to take us in with him so he would have more time to talk with us and help us with our homework.'

Di Bella was not, however, unreasonably demanding. In Adolfo's words, 'He believed the most important thing was that we should learn to study intelligently, learn to reason and to think for ourselves. People often talk about loving their children without understanding what that really means. His kind of love was unselfish. He gave us every opportunity to make the most of our talents, not just materially, that wasn't his concern. He wanted us to develop our own capabilities and talents to the best extent. For me, that's what loving your children is all about.'

Giuseppe, the first-born son (known as Pippo in the family), had a stricter upbringing than Adolfo. The professor was keen to look after every aspect of his intellectual development, and was forever buying him books to supplement his standard school texts. When he began to learn Greek his father decided to learn it too so that he could help him with his homework.

Giuseppe and his father are now also linked by professional bonds. He too chose medicine as his profession, and specialises in the study and treatment of tumours, using the professor's controversial techniques. He is convinced that the line of research initiated by his father is destined to become one of the most important breakthroughs in medical history.

The true inspirational force in Luigi Di Bella's life has undoubtedly been his wife Francesca. She was a traditional Sicilian woman and devoted her life to her

home and family. The warmth and happiness of family
life focused around her.

Christmas was the most important time of the year
for the Di Bella family; it was the only holiday that the
professor regularly observed. For a few days he would
forget his work and enjoy the atmosphere of domestic
bliss. The house was always full of gifts, not so much
from family members as from grateful patients, eager
to express their gratitude to a doctor who always
refused to be paid for his consultations.

It was only with his wife that Di Bella was able to
dismiss his professional problems and the antagonism
of his colleagues. In his many letters to her both
during and immediately after the war, when they were
separated because of his illness, he wrote of his
progress at the university and his fight against its
unwieldy, Byzantine bureaucracy. He often spoke to
her of his colleagues' envy. His wife tried to console
him and encouraged him to continue fighting for his
research. Optimistic by nature, she retained a profound
belief in her husband and refused to accept defeat,
even when the doctor himself felt the situation was
hopeless.

The death of Francesca, in 1992, was a terrible blow
for the entire family. The father and his sons flew from
Modena to Messina the moment they heard that
Francesca was unwell, but it was already too late. The
morning after her death, Di Bella walked to his father-
in-law's old house for a last look at the place where he
first courted his wife over fifty years previously.

University Life

The professor published numerous articles throughout the war, and his first findings on retinoids (vitamin A derivatives, which were later to play a significant role in his cancer research) come from that period. Paradoxically, the more he studied, the more he felt that his view (which already diverged from that of conventional science) was too narrowly focused, and that there were still many gaps in his knowledge. He wanted to understand personally all the concepts needed to develop new theories and cures, so he enrolled in the Faculty of Chemistry, and later in Pharmacology, at the University of Modena, earning two further degrees. In 1943, he began teaching physiology courses for students of natural sciences, biology and pharmacology, holding this teaching position until he retired in 1984.

'He was surrounded by very few friends and a large crowd of parasites,' Di Bella's son Adolfo says. 'Many of his colleagues just took advantage of him. They asked him to "look over" their work, which often meant rewriting it. I could name some names…Many of the people who benefited from his help are the same who criticised his work and later ridiculed him.'

At the end of the 1960s, Di Bella had a moment of inspiration which was to alter the direction of his cancer research for the rest of his career. His insights emerged from watching the slow death by leukaemia of a friend's seven-year-old son. From that moment on, he decided to dedicate his life to the search for a cure for cancer.

He first revealed his findings in 1969, when he presented his experimental results to the 45th Congress of the Italian Society for Experimental Biology in Sassari. His study, in laboratory rats, showed a marked increase in blood platelets (also called thrombocytes) after the ganglia (nerve tissue) of the *habenulae* (fibres connecting to an area of the brain called the thalamus) had been constantly stimulated for 72 hours. It confirmed the link he suspected between blood cancers and the central nervous system.

Throughout the 1960s and 1970s, relations between the professor and his colleagues in Modena had steadily worsened. Apart from a few close friends, most academics and doctors were wary of this brilliant scholar, infamous throughout the university for the awkward questions with which he confounded 'experts' during discussions and conferences. Many refused to give their lectures if they knew he was going to be in the audience. So determined were they to keep him away that some reportedly had Di Bella misinformed about the meetings being held.

The escalating hostility in the university towards the professor and his work eventually reached the point of no return when, on 6 December 1973, he was invited to speak at a conference of the Surgical Medicine Society of Bologna, presided over by Dr Domenico Campanacci, an internationally renowned clinician. During Di Bella's lecture, entitled 'Physiological perspectives in the treatment of haemopathies', he revealed that he had successfully cured seven cases of serious haematological (blood-related) illnesses. Among the cases presented, all of them meticulously documented, there was one of a boy suffering from leukaemia (an abnormal increase in white cells, or leucocytes, in blood and bone marrow) whose platelet count with this treatment was recorded to have risen from 7,000 to 50,000 in just ten days of treatment. There was such an awesome mass of research backing up his presentation that the medical community could only listen open-mouthed.*

The news was immediately taken up by the national newspapers, and subsequently by the world press. The bushy-haired scientist who claimed to have cured

---

* 'Physiological orientation in the treatment of haemopathies', L. Di Bella, annual conference of the Surgical Medicine Society of Bologna, 6 December 1973, published in Medical Sciences Bulletin, No. 1, 1974.

seven children of leukaemia with a new and revolutionary treatment had become internationally famous. The repercussions of his popularity with the press were immense: the resentment of his colleagues in some cases developed into open hostility and his life was even threatened.

Luigi Mele, a high-powered lawyer from Milan, met Di Bella in 1973 at the conference in Bologna. Heavily involved in politics, Mele later discussed the professor's startling research at length with the then Minister of Health, Vittorio Colombo. He mentioned the many patients who professed to have been completely cured by the novel treatment and the fact that the professor was successful in curing other illnesses besides cancer. The Minister listened with interest and Mele went on to hint at the international prestige that the Italian Health Service could attract if it collaborated with this exceptional doctor to promote his search for a viable cancer cure. But the Minister's response was: 'If they're roses, they'll bloom.' The subject was never brought up again, and Mele decided to leave politics soon after.*

In 1996 Mele himself developed skin cancer but, after three months of medication under Di Bella's care, the mole, and its associated malignancy, disappeared. Today, the lawyer devotes his free time to advising other cancer patients of their legal rights to follow the professor's therapy.

---

* Vittorio Colombo was Italian Minister of Health from 14 March to 22 November 1974.

After the press attention that Di Bella received, his hospital apparatus was sabotaged, and his laboratory animals poisoned. Many believe these violent acts are proof of a conspiracy against Di Bella's methods. It is possible that the hospital staff were intimidated by Di Bella's fierce intellect, and his refusal to accept compromise. Some felt that the faculty's image was suffering due to Di Bella's controversial contributions at conventions and medical congresses. Whatever the reason, there is no doubt that the constant sensational reports of the difficult cases which Di Bella reputedly cured put others in the shade.

The doctor became increasingly convinced that he needed a quiet place away from the antagonism and aggravation of the university environment to carry on with his research undisturbed. He scraped together as much money as he could, borrowed the rest, and managed to buy a small plot of land on the outskirts of Modena. He drew up the plans for the laboratory himself and even helped to construct it, shovel in hand. 'I managed to break the wheelbarrow with all the cement I moved in it,' he recalls, laughing. Here, in this laboratory, which also houses consulting rooms, Di Bella was finally able to work and see his patients in peace.

A Selfless Teacher

In marked contrast to his relationship with his colleagues, Di Bella was immensely popular with his students. In all his years of teaching, the doctor was absent from his lectures only once – in order to pay his last respects to his sister.

The professor's popularity can be inferred by the fact that he was the only lecturer permitted to enter the university during the student sit-ins of 1968. There is a certain irony in the fact that this small, unassuming and quietly determined man has managed to achieve in 1998 what all those impassioned medical students thirty years ago could not: to storm the bastions of education and health care and expose them to public scrutiny.

Anna Piccagli, one of Di Bella's ex-students during the period of the 1968 demonstrations, explains why the students allowed him to cross the barricades when all his colleagues were categorically denied access. 'Students know whether or not a teacher is sincere;

they are often the most severe critics. Di Bella
certainly was not ambitious for himself, and was
uninterested in both money and prestige. We liked that
in him.' His pupils admired him, she thinks, for his
dedication to his work, the enthusiasm he was able to
transmit, and for his uncompromising fairness. 'If you
knew your stuff, he passed you; if you didn't, he failed
you — it was as simple as that.' There was no
favouritism. He was also known to keep an eye on
students from poorer backgrounds, and tried to help
them find jobs when he could.

'There were other very good teachers, but none
who were able to go into their subject-matter at the
level of detail that he could and still make you
understand the material. Sometimes he substituted for
other teachers in different areas of study, and his
lectures were always much more interesting and
engaging. I suppose that created a lot of envy among
the staff. Perhaps they were afraid he'd push them all
out of a job.'

Some of Di Bella's most devoted students went on
to achieve considerable professional success. Dr Achille
Norsa, now a successful surgical consultant in the
Cardiovascular and Thoracic Department at the
Ospedale Maggiore in Verona, is a strong supporter of
his ex-professor. Norsa has been experimenting under
Di Bella's guidance since 1995, when the professor's
tumour research first came to his attention. He uses
new treatments for thoracic neoplasias (tumours)
which combine advanced surgical techniques with

MDB (Di Bella's Multi-Therapy). Norsa is currently one of the practitioners most experienced in applying MDB treatment.

'It was 1961, and I was in my second year of medical studies at Modena when I started the human physiology course,' he remembers. 'I was fascinated by physiology, which seemed to open up the secrets of life itself. There was one teacher in the department whom I found particularly interesting. He was a modest, grandfatherly kind of chap. I remember he had a shock of white hair and rode to the lecture hall on an old, rickety bicycle. But, in reality, he was a real anti-conformist. His lectures were fascinating; we all listened with rapt attention when he spoke. He was one of those rare teachers who manage to keep his pupils' interest at maximum level all the time. What he said was always carefully thought out, clear and concise – there was none of that woolly vagueness which university lecturers seem to like and often resort to.'

This much-praised professor was Luigi Di Bella, who had already become a legendary figure in the university by this early date. He was regarded by students as a brilliant scientist but also a loner and an eccentric.

Norsa continues, 'I remember that we used to joke among ourselves that he'd discovered a synthetic food which he lived on, since no-one had ever seen him eat or drink. Passing by the windows of his study on my way home, I saw that the lights were always on, even in the middle of the night. That is when I realised how dedicated he was to his work. After 1966, when I graduated in medicine and decided to specialise in surgery, I left Modena and lost touch with the professor. But the enthusiasm that he transmitted for physiology and for the study of biological systems never left me.'

Norsa now dedicates himself to cancer research and addresses the problems in finding a cure. 'I think one of the greatest difficulties facing us in our fight against cancer is the strict division between scientific specialties, and the lack of communication between experts working in different fields. Cancer is an extremely wide-ranging medical problem which is still, for the most part, unresolved because it is not a simple biological phenomenon. It involves very complex mechanisms and systems that we do not yet really understand. Surgery is one of the few available options, but none will claim that it suffices on its own. Above all, a thorough knowledge of these systems requires far-reaching preparation in more fields than one, the type of extensive knowledge that an individual scientist rarely possesses. Surgery, oncology, radiology, immunology – they all have a role to play in obtaining the complete picture. Physiology, however, is the discipline which underpins all of these specialties; it is, undoubtedly, the key to our under-standing the disease.'

A few years ago, Norsa heard that a family friend had been successfully cured of a tumour by Di Bella.

He called the professor to discuss the case. When they met in Modena, over three decades after their last encounter, Norsa found that the professor's penetrating mind was as sharp as ever and his speech as fluent. It was Norsa who had some difficulty following the older man's theories, because he had not kept up with advances in Di Bella's research into tumour pathology. Norsa was convinced that Di Bella was on to something of fundamental importance. Fired up once again by the enthusiasm of his former teacher, Norsa immediately set about filling in the gaps in his knowledge of cancer research.

That meeting proved to be the first of many. The professor offered to let Norsa document the progress of the cases he was currently treating, and passed him the documents detailing his therapy. It was immediately apparent to Norsa that positive results were coming out of this carefully balanced treatment. The evidence in the patients' clinical records was clear. 'I had never seen such encouraging results in cancer treatment, neither from chemotherapy nor radiotherapy,' says Norsa. 'I started thinking that we could probably improve the odds even further if we combined his MDB therapy with the surgical techniques I had been using.' Di Bella agreed to collaborate with Norsa on condition that the surgical intervention be strictly monitored.

Time and again Norsa saw the treatment yield positive results. In one case, the patient's cancer went into remission only a few months after a complicated lung operation. The professor was delighted, but not unduly surprised. 'I was able to document the case with x-rays and biopsies, and the results were undeniable,' comments Norsa. 'I also kept detailed records of fifty other cases that we treated over a period of one year and, although I admit that it is not a long enough period to document definitive remission properly, I noted the apparent success of this "surgical-biological therapy" (as the professor calls it) in at least four other cases. In general, there was a significant improvement in the patients' conditions, though this was less significant in pre-terminal cases, or after prolonged chemo- or radiotherapy. More importantly, with this treatment the patient's suffering seemed to be considerably lessened and, in terminal cases, death came in a much more dignified way. I feel privileged to have had the chance to work with Di Bella, and to have made a contribution to the development of his therapy. He's not really a religious man but I'll always remember something he said to me: "I thank God for helping me understand, through suffering, the meaning of life." I think if anyone understands the essence of human life, he does.'

Another of Di Bella's ex-students, Maria Teresa Rossi (known as Deda), was hired by the doctor as his research assistant in 1966. While still a student, Deda had approached the professor to discuss a particularly serious case – her own. She had been diagnosed with lupus erythematosus (an inflammatory disease of the skin and internal body systems), and the prognosis was not promising – her doctors predicted that she would have two years at most to live. Di Bella, in a later account of his relationship with this remarkable woman, wrote: 'She asked me to clarify her diagnosis with a simplicity which I found touching. She listened attentively while I tried to explain her condition. Her face was swollen and misshapen from the cortisone she'd been prescribed.' The middle-aged professor took the young woman under his wing; she soon came to represent for him the daughter he had never had.

Di Bella began to treat her illness, and she made encouraging progress. She dedicated 22 years of her life as his most trusted assistant. She was an enthusiastic and conscientious researcher, fired by the same thirst for knowledge and will to help the suffering which motivated the professor himself. Before her death in 1988, she reached the position of Associate Professor of General Physiology in the Pharmacology Faculty of the University of Modena.

When Deda died, the professor was overcome with grief. He ate almost nothing for a month, and hardly spoke to anyone. In order to lessen his sense of loss, he covered the walls of his home with photographs of his favourite protégée. 'We shared so much,' Di Bella says sadly, 'Things you can't express in words. She saw me break down and cry once when the mother of a six-year-old recited a list of her beloved child's new skills rather than describe the relentless development of the tumour which was threatening her life. Another time, we both wept when a little three-year-old, blind from leukaemia, sang to us over the phone; he was so delighted to be home after spending many months in hospital.'

Professor Di Bella is a deeply spiritual man; something spurs him to make the journey every Sunday morning, before beginning his day's work, to the little cemetery at Fanano where Deda is buried. This year, the Italian Association for Cancer Patients was established to bring together those treated by the professor. At his request, it was named after Maria Teresa Rossi.

Another ex-student of Di Bella's, Barbara Palladini, studied physiology under his instruction, and was due to take her final exam the year before he retired. Unfortunately, she was involved in a serious accident shortly beforehand: 90% of her body was covered with burns. During the oral exam, Di Bella spoke to her kindly, and allowed her to remain seated (it is usual for students to stand throughout), but made no other outward sign of concession to her condition. He then proceeded to question her, not about what she had studied in her textbooks, but about what had happened after her accident. He asked her opinions about her physical condition, the changes to which her body had been subjected and the chemical exchanges which had taken place at a cellular level. He asked her to talk about oedema (accumulation of fluid in tissue), and about the reasons why a burn victim requires 10,000 calories a day instead of the 2,000 of a healthy person (because the amount of carbohydrate stored as glycogen in the liver increases), and about the effect of shock on the lungs. At the end of the exam, she realised that, via the unusual format in which he had chosen to test her, he had also given her a great deal of useful medical advice.

The professor's vast knowledge of a number of fields, and his consequent overview of associated drug complications, has made him an authority not just for medical students, but also for pharmacists, who often refer to him for his opinion on chemical substances and their possible side effects. Di Bella has taught 'pure' physiology to a great many pharmacists. He is eager to lend his expertise to those in the field, since he is particularly interested in the the dangers of pharmaceuticals being prescribed without full awareness of their potential effects on the patient. One of the first professionals to publicly speak out in support of Di Bella was not a doctor, but a pharmacist who had followed the professor's work on the importance of galenical (plant-based) and magisterial (unusual remedies specially prescribed by a physician) substances, particularly vitamins and the hormone melatonin.

So many of Di Bella's students recall his exhaustive knowledge of every aspect of his subject, and the incredible enthusiasm he engendered during his lectures. His classes were famous in the university for running well over time. At the end of his lessons there were always people who stayed behind to ask questions, and the professor never turned them away.

Vigildo Ferrari, now 74 years old, comes from Gonzaga, near Mantua. At the end of the Second World War, he decided to enrol in the University of Modena. He admired Di Bella's lectures on human physiology and biochemistry, claiming that the professor was 'able to explain things that we couldn't find in any textbook. He had a real gift for presenting his subject with a sort of mathematical clarity which made it accessible to everyone.' In 1946, Ferrari applied to become an intern in physiology and prepared his thesis under the professor's direction. He remained with his mentor until 1955, during which time he also studied chemistry, which Di Bella advised as the only way to broaden his horizons.

Di Bella had an excellent research group during this period: all those who participated were later successful in their chosen professions. They were expected to work hard under his direction, but he treated them fairly, asking nothing that he would not have been prepared to do himself. 'He was like a father to us,' Ferrari recounts. The professor's team met on Saturdays. Each student was required to be familiar with their fellow classmates' studies, and to give a report on their own progress to date. The group worked well together as they were convinced that their projects would have important future repercussions. It was only when Di Bella's post in the department was discontinued some years later, that the group sadly broke up. 'If I am forced to leave, you will all be forced out too,' he had warned them early on in their collaboration. His words proved prophetic.

Ferrari went on to teach chemistry at technical high schools until the professor, who never forgot his more gifted students, called him with news of a pharmacist's position in a town near Mantua. The doctor advised him to look out for the exam announcement in the local paper, 'because everything here is going from bad to worse, and at least this job will give you the chance to earn a living'. Ferrari took the exam and won first place.

The student and teacher continued to see each other whenever possible, and the pharmacist sometimes lent Di Bella a hand, teaching at the university. 'I just couldn't forget the man,' Ferrari confesses. 'If you work with him, you feel you are a "real" scientist, and that what you are doing is relevant. He is inspiring.'

Ferrari remembers the professor not only as a scientific genius but also as a demanding teacher and inflexible moralist. He relates the story of how Di Bella was infuriated at receiving a letter of recommendation from the Minister of Education, with a request to find his grandson a post within the university. It turned out that this well-connected candidate was unable to calculate the decimals in an exam question on red blood cells. 'The professor was speechless. He took it as an affront that a university graduate could be stumped by such a simple calcula-tion. He failed the boy immediately, saying "forwarding incompetent people just causes more problems. If he was at least capable of reasoning it might be another story, but in this case…out he goes."'

At the time that Di Bella first started to use the hormone melatonin in his treatments, Ferrari had taken over a pharmacy with a laboratory attached, in Bologna. He was aware that the professor had been studying melatonin for some time, and so when his mentor asked him to start producing melatonin because his patients would be needing it, Ferrari set to it – he had already been making the pure vitamin form used by Di Bella for some years. Today, Ferrari's chemical laboratory cannot keep up with the demand. He shrugs, 'I've given the exact formula for melatonin to the Ministry of Health, because I can't cope on my own any more,' he explains. 'The Ministry has excellent laboratories at their disposal; they should be doing it. All they need is the will and guaranteed, high-quality materials.'

The professor's influence is also tangible in a pharmacy in Modena, just a short walk from his consulting room. It belongs to the Palladini family, pharmacists since the last century. Today it is run by sisters Isabella and Maria, and Maria's daughter Barbara, all of whom qualified under him and remember the man and his teaching vividly.

In 1969, Isabella, then a young graduate, was invited by Di Bella to take up the position of Assistant Professor in Human Physiology. Whenever she was in difficulty with an academic problem, whether relating to chemistry, physics or maths, the professor was always ready and able to assist her. At the time, he was also absorbed in translating scientific articles from German (which he learned during the war), saying that the information published in Italian textbooks was hopelessly out of date, and that all the important research work was currently being done abroad. Isabella, like most of those who have known the professor well, believes he is both an extraordinary human being and an exceptional scientist. 'He has absolutely no interest in making money from his work,' she says. 'He is a truly selfless person. I would even go as far as to compare him to Mother Teresa of Calcutta.'

She recounts a famous incident about the professor in order to support her rather extreme viewpoint. In the 1950s, a big pharmaceutical company telephoned him about a problem they were having with the insulin they produced. The insulin seemed to be gradually losing its effectiveness and many customers were complaining. Di Bella traced the problem to the presence of a microscopic fungus which had infiltrated the packaging. He had unknowingly provided the company with a faultless, 'official' solution, enabling them to avoid huge financial losses, a ruined reputation and legal action. The professor refused to accept the blank cheque offered him by the grateful directors of the company, accepting instead a small MV98 moped which he thought might be useful for getting to work and back when the weather prevented him from using his bike. He later donated it to his needy students and returned to using his rickety old bicycle.

Isabella claims to have personally seen many of Di Bella's patients recover. 'They come here to refill their prescriptions for the drugs he uses in the cure. That seems like evidence to me." Her sister Maria tells how she spent her Easter vacation one year at the university, taking the professor's famous cramming course for students who had missed lessons. 'It was an unforgettable experience,' she enthuses. 'It really opened up my horizons.' Di Bella helped her in every way possible, explaining the best methods of study, where to find appropriate texts, which material she could omit, and so on.

'The ultimate goal of his method was always to encourage students to reason for themselves,' she says. 'Those studying with him had to work hard, but the discipline and study strategies we learned remained with us throughout our careers.' Maria feels that Di Bella is also a truly gifted physician, with an exceptional ability to observe the human body and diagnose illnesses accurately. 'He will look at the skin's texture, the skin beneath the eyes, the irises, whether the eyes are swollen or not. He'll take the patient's blood pressure in different places and at different times throughout the day – he's very aware of how important it is to repeat these checks regularly in order to get the complete picture.' His dedication to humanity and to science is total and the cases he treats and studies are frequently difficult ones which other specialists are unable to resolve.

Di Bella has spent most of his time teaching and advancing his research at the university's Physiology Institute, but he never stopped seeing patients. It came as no surprise to Di Bella's patients or ex-students when, in 1990, he received a 'kindness prize' from the Catholic Church in recognition of his altruism in treating patients free of charge.

The Crucial Years

From 1970 to 1974 Di Bella and his assistant Maria
Teresa Rossi (nicknamed Deda) began to experiment
with the use of melatonin. The professor first used the
hormone on himself, administering high doses of
soluble melatonin into his own bloodstream, without
any side effects. They then used it in treating patients
suffering from both solid tumours and leukaemia. The
initial results were encouraging. The application of the
therapy to cases of thalassaemia (a severe, inherited
form of anaemia) showed good results, promoting the
patients' general recovery without recourse to blood
transfusion. 'Use in cases of gastric carcinoma and
Hodgkin's disease (a cancer-related illness involving
enlarged lmph nodes, spleen and liver, and anaemia)
confirmed the absence of toxicity, and underlined the
real potential of melatonin,' Professor Di Bella
declared. 'Malignant cancer tumours could be cured
too,' he claimed, 'if the substance is administered
together with vitamins and growth factor inhibitors.'

In 1973, he introduced melatonin into the treatment of patients suffering from sub-acute and chronic lymphatic leukaemia (a sharp increase in lymphocytes, a type of leucocyte, or white cell, produced by the lymph nodes, in blood and bone marrow) and essential thrombocytopenia (a reduction in blood platelets). Many of the patients are still alive and well today. Dr Di Bella believes that melatonin by itself has no measurable effect on cancer cells but, in synergy with other substances, it is capable of saving lives.*

In January 1974, the professor attended the 26th International Congress of Physiological Sciences in New Delhi, where he presented an extremely well-received paper entitled 'Nervous control of thrombo-cytopoiesis' (i.e. platelet formation) that was to have further important international repercussions. In 1976, he explained his anti-cancer therapy at the 16th World Congress of Haematology in Kyoto and, in 1977, he participated in the International Congress on the Pineal Gland organised by Isaac Nir of the Pharmacology Department of the Hadassah Medical Center of Jerusalem.

Over the next ten years, Di Bella divided his time between teaching, seeing patients and conducting

---

* Numerous articles have been published about melatonin and
  its possible applications in anti-tumour therapies. Of
  particular interest is 'The validity of melatonin as an
  oncostatic agent', A. Pauzer, M.Viljoen, (Department of
  Physiology, University of Pretoria, South Africa), Journal of

experimental studies on his innovative theory of cancer treatment. He worked incessantly, devoting seven days a week to his passion, or 'calling' (as he sometimes describes it) to alleviate human suffering. The professor believes that the key to improving treatment outcomes is better education about cancer prevention and treatment, especially for those entering into the health field.

In 1984, the professor retired from his teaching position, at the age of 72, in order to spend more time on research. At the end of 1989, the news was leaked to the press that he had been short-listed for the Nobel Prize.

Over the next eight years, Di Bella was left to work alone, and in relative peace. By 1997, his name was well known – and spoken in hushed tones – within a closed circle of academics and doctors. The word of mouth among the Italian population, however, had already passed judgement, and the doctor had more patients than he could handle. The ingredients were all there for a media circus, but no one could have possibly predicted the extent of the furore to come.

In June 1997, at a conference in Bologna, Luigi Di Bella's son, Dr Giuseppe Di Bella, delivered a paper on his father's work to an audience of physicians and oncologists (cancer specialists) of international standing. It proved to be a controversial meeting in many respects, and the heated reactions to details of the now famous 'Di Bella cure' resounded worldwide.

One of the doctors present, the famous French

oncologist Phillipe Lagard, admitted in his own presentation, 'We cannot even be sure whether the few cancer patients apparently cured by chemotherapy would have recovered in any case if submitted to different sorts of treatment'. He expressed disappointment in the lack of current research initiatives and of accomplished scientists and researchers in the field; he also criticised heavily the teaching methods in European medical faculties:'...so far no-one has come up with a viable solution, but then look at the way we are currently training new doctors – it simply isn't working. I speak to young medics in the university and I'm shocked by what they say – it's obvious they have no idea what they're talking about.'*

Many in the audience nodded in agreement. At the same forum, the Florentine biochemist, Gianfranco Pantellini launched a savage indictment of the pharmaceutical industry, which he said 'can no longer be differentiated from that of petro-chemicals, arms or telecommunications...with drastic consequences for research in the seemingly unrewarding field of oncology.'**

Although little press coverage was given to the conference, the issues raised there predicted the direction the discussion of cancer research and treatment was about to take in the public sphere. The 'Di Bella affair' proved to be not just a transient news

---

* 11th Fiera della Salute, Bazzano, Bologna, 21–29 June 1997
** Ibid.

story, but central to a number of bitter controversies regarding the integrity of the medical profession. The exposure of the enormous financial interests behind the long-standing promotion of conventional therapies triggered a surge of public outrage and critical attention which still continues.

In early July 1997, Luigi Di Bella presented to the World Congress of Physiology in St Petersburg the results of his research on citocalsine, a retinoid substance which he is currently studying and which he suggests may hold the key to a cure for AIDS, among other illnesses.

Later that month, in Rome, the professor held a national conference entitled 'Cancer: Old Aspects, New Treatments', aimed at medical experts, many of whom had always vilified him. The audience consisted of 336 doctors, 50 pharmacists, and 70 journalists. Although many authoritative figures invited failed to attend, journalists from the major daily newspapers were present. During the conference, Di Bella presented his MDB (Di Bella's Multi -Therapy) clearly and convincingly to the audience. He spoke with the lucidity and enthusiasm of a teacher entranced by his subject. Despite his age – 85 – he stood on the platform at length explaining the results of thirty years of research. After three straight hours of lecturing, Di Bella turned to his audience: 'Now, if you're not all too tired', he said innocently, 'I'd like to explain another few related points...' He was encouraged by approving applause from the floor. The audience loved him.

The two-day conference contributed a great deal to establishing the professor's popularity with the public. It had become clear that the world owed a debt to this unassuming doctor whose obstinate dedication to his work, in the face of hostility and ridicule, had the potential to benefit many. The spirit of his presentation was summed up by the conference chairman's conclusion: 'We can successfully defeat this disease only if we make that quantum leap of the imagination which will enable us to look anew at the drugs we already have available, and to devise new ways of combining and administering them according to sound scientific principles and meticulous research...*

In October 1997, doctors from all over Italy came to attend a seminar held by Di Bella and organised by the National Association of Families against Cancer, in Fanano, a town in the mountains near Modena. Many of the professionals interviewed afterwards said they were fascinated by the therapeutic possibilities raised by the maverick scientist who spoke to them for two solid days about the composition of MDB and its applications.

The professor himself was somewhat less enthusiastic about his audience. 'It's discouraging to realise that I've just explained, for the umpteenth time, basic concepts which all doctors should remember from medical school. Vitamin biochemistry and

---

* Associazione Italiana Assistenza Malati Neoplastici (AIAMN) Conference, Rome, 17–18 July 1997

cellular physiology are fundamental subjects which should be taught in every medical faculty in the country. The way medicine is studied today is inadequate... The final word on the exact composition of my treatment (MDB), and the dosage of each substance used, is left to the discretion of the physician. But in order to apply the therapy properly, he or she must be able to assess the individual patient's condition accurately, 100% accurately. That is where our problems lie, not in the therapy itself.'

When the convention ended, Adolfo Di Bella greeted some of the faces he recognised in the crowd. One of the doctors said, 'I came because we – myself, my colleagues and our hospital director – are all tired of seeing cancer patients dying like flies. I, personally, must have seen over five thousand patients die. It's a holocaust. But I've met some of the patients treated by your father, and their recovery is remarkable; they seem able to lead normal lives again. Finally, it looks like you might have given us a ray of hope.'

Another oncologist approached the professor to confess, sadly, 'I have been unable to sleep for three months, thinking about all those people I sent to their deaths over the past twenty years when MDB therapy already existed. If only I had known.'

A physician from Padua relates how he followed Di Bella's treatment when he himself was diagnosed with Hodgkin's disease. After successfully curing himself, he began prescribing the treatment for his patients.

Conspicuous by their absence at this convention

however, were the hordes of pharmaceutical company representatives usually found behind the stacks of enticing freebies they use to wangle their way into the good graces of attending doctors. Neither were there any at the professor's Rome conference, as they know they are unwelcome when he speaks.

Di Bella's seminar at Fanano was described in the press by those attending as 'revolutionary' and 'fascinating'. His skillful presentation the basic concepts of cell and tissue physiology fundamental to the development of his therapy was judged to be masterly. The discussions appealed to public curiousity, and many began asking about Di Bella's controversial treatment. The professor's philosophical approach to curing cancer, his alternative cancer treatment, and his gentle, altruistic manner struck a cord with the Italian public, as it was soon to do internationally.

In fact, in January 1998, Di Bella was invited to Brussels to explain his anti-cancer treatment to the European parliament.* There, he caused a storm when he declared that his therapy was also effective in patients with multiple sclerosis and Alzheimer's disease. With his extensive knowledge of the physiology of the nervous system, he claims to have successfully treated other neurological diseases as well.

In Brussels, he told a group of international reporters how his life had been threatened, both recently and in

---

* Presentation on MDB to officials of European Parliament,
  Brussels, 28 January 1998

the past because his findings exclude the use of chemotherapy, thus raising the question of just how far the medical community and the pharmaceutical industry will go to protect their lucrative and intertwined interests. In 1996, while returning home one evening on his bicycle, Di Bella was suddenly hit on the head. He lost consciousness, and woke up in hospital. The blow has seriously damaged his hearing in one ear. He filed a report with the police, but the case was never solved. There were other strange and threatening incidents too, like the time in the summer of 1974 when he became desperately ill after drinking bottled water which he kept in the refrigerator of the university's Physiology Department. Fortunately, he recovered, but when it happened a second time he decided to have the water analysed. It contained significant quantities of phosphoric esters.

He had been poisoned.

The Cure

An Alternative

Cancer: A general term for more than 100 diseases in which abnormal cells grow out of control and form malignant tumours. Tumours occur when the cells of a tissue or organ multiply in an uncontrolled fashion unrelated to the biological requirements of the body and not to meet the needs of repair or of normal replacement. In contrast to benign tumours, which enlarge in a specific place, and cause damage by pressure on adjacent tissues, malignant tumours invade, destroy and spread to other tissues. The cells of a malignant tumour may also be carried in the blood stream and lymphatics, and lodge in distant organs where they continue to spread and enlarge (metastases). Cancer kills by destroying vital tissues, by interfering with the performance of their functions through ulceration, bleeding and infection, and by affecting bodily nutrition.

The Barnes & Noble Encyclopedia

Despite decades of research, the reasons why cancers develop are still largely unknown, and Di Bella believes it will probably be years before science is able to solve this mystery. A sudden insight while witnessing a child's death from leukaemia caused Di Bella to search for a treatment which focused on the inhibition of cancer cells' proliferation, as opposed to their destruction. Despite the dreadful reputation of the disease, the fear it inspires in both patients and doctors, and the daunting degree of ignorance about its cause which still exists in the scientific community, he decided many years ago to accept the the challenge of finding a cure for cancer.

A malignant tumour is a threatening and destructive growth, which intrudes on the cellular life cycle, suffocating it, like weeds in a flower garden. But, as a physiologist, Di Bella views the tumour as a life form – lethal, but nonetheless living. It is therefore regulated by the same principles as all other living things. In order to conquer the disease, he advocates a return to basic concepts underpinning the complex and intriguing mechanisms that regulate life itself.

Normal tumour development is almost always caused by alterations in the dynamics of cellular growth patterns. According to Di Bella, by manipulating tumour cell growth (an essential process in the very biogenesis of life), one can eventually achieve one of the key objectives in the fight against cancer: the suppression the growth of tumour cells through cellular 'old age' and their spontaneous physiological degeneration. Limited, and harmless, quantities of substances that discourage tumour cell growth, if administered quickly enough, can accelerate the process of apoptosis (cell breakdown) to the point where the cancer can be brought under control and the patient, although still affected by the disease, can begin to lead a normal life again.

Approaching the study of tumours as a physiologist with wide-ranging expertise in the fields of physics, organic and inorganic chemistry, thermodynamics and biochemistry, Di Bella has made significant discoveries relating to cell development and the interaction on a cellular level of the nervous, endocrine and cardio-vascular systems. He regards physiology as a vital means of explaining living phenomena. 'A doctor's knowledge should embrace all aspects of physiology and clinical medicine. Extreme specialisation is, in my opinion, a mistake. Nowadays, patients with the most minor complaints are sent from one specialist to another; each expert provides a different, contra-dictory opinion, which results in total confusion. It seems as though medical professionals can no longer find common ground in their opinions, treatments or diagnoses.'

The anti-cancer Multi-Therapy (MDB) developed by Di Bella during years of painstaking research represents a complete turnaround with respect to the treatments traditionally prescribed. The personalisa-tion of the treatment, and Di Bella's idea of treating the person as a whole (and not just the tumour) is an important factor that, oddly enough, became 'out-dated' in modern medicine's drive towards special-isation.

In modern cancer treatment, each specialist diagnoses and treats the element (the tumour, the heart, the blood etc.) pertaining to his or her special-isation. MDB insists on an alternative to 'modern' treatment by addressing the whole organism (i.e. the patient). The professor has always believed in what is now popularly called 'holistic' health and medicine.

'Standard' cancer therapy is based almost exclusively on three main methods: surgery, radiotherapy and chemotherapy. The objective of these approaches is to either physically remove, attack or kill the affected cells, thereby curing the patient.

Chemotherapy, the administration of a cocktail of cytotoxic (cell–destroying) drugs, was introduced after the Second World War at a time when these substances were being studied for their destructive action. Chemotherapy originates with the idea of aggressive intervention against cancer, which most experts now agree has limited value.

Although designed to attack primarily the rapidly growing cells of a tumour, these poisonous substances cannot differentiate; they also destroy normal cells at one or more points in their life cycle. The fast-growing cells most likely to be affected are blood cells forming in the bone marrow and the cells in the digestive tract, reproductive system and hair follicles. Chemotherapy affects the bone marrow's ability to make platelets, white blood cells (leucocytes) and red blood cells (erythrocytes), crucial elements in the immune system. As an effect of this damage, the patient suffers reduced resistance to infection, loss of hair, and sterility, among other problems. Anti-cancer drugs can also damage cells of the heart, kidney, bladder, lungs and nervous system.

Di Bella, however, believes that attacking the cancer cell, as in traditional therapies, should not be the objective of treatment, because elements capable of destroying cancer cells can also wipe out healthy cells. His approach, in contrast to that of chemotherapy, is therefore directed towards the processes responsible for the formation and growth of the cancer cell, and is crucially aimed at reinforcing the body's capacity to obstruct the reproduction of diseased cells. He arrests tumour cells' growth by creating biological conditions hostile to their proliferation and conducive to their destruction. With his therapy, the greatest anti-tumour effect results directly from the body's own strengthened immune system.

The elements administered in MDB create conditions under which cancer cells are unable to grow or reproduce. According to Di Bella's findings, it takes very little to obtain the changes in the biological environment capable of causing a significant reduction in tumour mass, so, with his approach, doctors are able to control the anomalous processes of cancer cells without poisoning the rest of the body. With chemo-therapy, in contrast, tumour cells often begin to

reproduce immediately after chemotherapy is suspended, while, with MDB, cancer cells self-destruct
permanently, leaving healthy cells unharmed.

Di Bella is not against the use of chemotherapy in
itself, but he opposes the traditional view of this
drastic treatment as the only means of curing cancer.
He questions the duration of chemotherapy, the
method used to administer it (intravenously) and the
high dosages regularly prescribed. Both Di Bella
himself and his followers are willing to prescribe
mainstream chemotherapy drugs, (hydroxyurea and
cyclophosphamide) for patients with cancer that is
actively proliferating. However, in contrast to their use
in orthodox chemotherapy, 'Di Bellians' prescribe
these two heavy-duty substances in tiny doses, to be
taken orally, and for short periods, depending on the
phase of tumour development and the capacity of the
individual patient to tolerate their toxicity. In addition,
Di Bella's method always complements the
administration of these two drugs with other
substances that protect healthy cell structure and the
immune system.

Neither does the professor dismiss on principle the
use of radiotherapy or surgery. He believes that both
applications play an important role in the treatment of
selected types of cancer. Radiotherapy, for instance,
can prove effective, if used sparingly, and at given
stages in the development of some tumours, while
surgery can be used to remove localised tumours.
'Every method has a certain value,' he explains.

'Surgery allows us to physically remove the affected tissue so that the cancer cells cannot spread to other parts of the body. It is the oldest method we know. Radiotherapy has a considerable capacity to destroy abnormal tissue...'

Radiotherapy is the use of radiation to treat malignant tumours. The radiation is usually directed in a beam from several different angles and carefully aimed so that the tumour receives the maximum concentration of x-rays. Alternatively, radioactive materials can be directly implanted into the tumour. The side effects of radiotherapy, however, are significant.

Di Bella has chosen to distance himself from these traditional treatments because he feels that they do not produce 'convincing enough" results. 'Each time invasive, chemo- or radiotherapy is used, there is a little more damage done to the whole organism. Over time, this secondary damage can ultimately lead to the death of the patient. In any case, the effect they produce is often temporary and their success rate varies widely from one patient to another, according to the type of tumour treated, the resistance of the individual, the way in which the therapy is applied, and the time elapsed from the original diagnosis to the actual application of the treatment. All of these variables should serve to underline the fact that we must be extremely wary of making generalisations about the possible dangers or benefits, effectiveness or destructiveness of any treatment methods.'

The professor finds it deeply distressing that the

majority of doctors advocate chemotherapy, and strongly believes that a combination of ignorance and financial interest are responsible for many such decisions.

The Tetralogy

Di Bella's Multi-Therapy (MDB), as explained previously, aims to reduce the proliferation of cancer cells while respecting the integrity of the rest of the body. The professor often refers to MDB as a 'tetralogy', since it consists of four main elements (melatonin, somatostatin, retinoids and bromo-criptine), substances already thoroughly tested and currently available in hospitals and pharmacies. These elements are taken at high doses and always in combination, as none of them displays anti-cancer activity when prescribed on its own.

The first element is **melatonin**, a hormone produced by the pineal gland,★ situated in the hypothalamus region of the brain. Di Bella claims that,

★ There are several articles on the relationship between dysfunction of the pineal gland, altered levels of melatonin in the body and the incidence of breast cancer. Of special interest is: 'The fountain of youth', W. Pierpaoli, WE. Regelson, *The Lancet*, 1978.

while melatonin alone cannot cure cancer, cancer cannot be cured without it.

The second element, **somatostatin**, relates to growth. Given that cancer cells grow just as healthy ones do, Di Bella asserts that it is possible to intervene to slow this process and eventually block it completely by the use of somatostatin, a hormone capable of inhibiting the action of growth hormone, among others, thereby reducing the rate of cellular development.

The third consists of **retinoids**, which include natural vitamin A and its esters and synthetic analogues. These substances are administered in conjunction with vitamin E, which increases their effectiveness.

The fourth element is **bromocriptine**, a drug that inhibits another growth substance, prolactin. It is inexpensive and available on prescription.

Often, MDB treatment is prescribed with the addition of the following substances given in varying combinations, depending on the type of tumour and its location, the patient's medical history and the specific symptoms that the individual case presents:

> adrenocorticotrophic hormone (ACTH)
> calcium salts
> potassium
> vitamin B1
> vitamin B6
> vitamin C
> vitamin D3

vagolytics or sympatholytics (inhibit muscle contraction and glandular secretions),

glucosamine (form of body sugar)

polygalacturonase (enzyme)

chondrosamine (form of body sugar)

liposomes (microscopic lipid sacs)

bile acids

hepatoprotectors (protect the liver)

integrators (encourage metabolism of substances administered)

In some cases, as mentioned previously, very small amounts of hydroxyurea and cyclophosphamide (two of the drugs used in traditional chemotherapy) are also prescribed.

MDB can be used effectively for most types of tumours (depending on the stage they have reached) by 'carefully calibrating [adjusting the doses of] the basic components of the therapy.'

Melatonin

In 1958, the American dermatologist A.B. Lerner, at the Yale University School of Medicine in Connecticut, was the first to isolate from the brain a white substance called melatonin.

Melatonin is derived from tryptophan, an amino acid widely found in proteins and essential for human metabolism. The highly complex transformation of tryptophan into melatonin takes place, in a series of phases and at varying speeds, in many of the body's organs, starting with the pineal gland. Once produced, melatonin is distributed throughout the body via the bloodstream where it is present in the plasma (the fluid in which blood cells are suspended) or the platelets. It later amalgamates with substances in the liver (sulphates and glycuronates) and is eventually eliminated in the saliva or urine.

In its voyage through the human anatomy melatonin performs many different functions (involving cells, nerve endings and hormone levels), with implications for the whole body. As it interacts with other chemical mediators and receptors, it is often referred to as being 'multidisciplinary'.

Melatonin uses its exceptional solubility, in the tiny space between the platelets and the endothelium (lining) of the capillaries, to regulate the chemical exchanges between the blood and the surrounding tissues. Melatonin plays an important role in maintaining cellular chain reactions, fundamental to sustaining life.

Eighteen years after it was discovered, a study was conducted to test whether taking melatonin could be harmful. A massive dose of 6.6 grams a day showed no significant signs of toxicity in humans, even when the treatment was continued for 35 consecutive days. A follow-up study of a patient who had received 250 milligrams intravenously for 7 days, still a very high dose, gave no indication of delayed toxicity years later.

These data convinced the doctors conducting the studies that melatonin could be used safely in clinical medicine. In fact, thousands of people have been taking it regularly for years, some under medical supervision and others for its supposed beneficial effects on their general health, without any significant reports of toxic effects. 'The reasons for this extreme tolerance to melatonin,' says Di Bella, 'are simple. Melatonin is derived from an amino acid, tryptophan. The reactions necessary to effect its conversion seem clear: they occur in cells which carry out extremely important functions, and they do not appear to produce toxic substances, perhaps because the amounts involved are so small. Melatonin and its precursor, serotonin, accumulate in high concentrations in the blood platelets and thromboblasts (cells where the platelets originate). This means it is unlikely for melatonin or serotonin to accumulate in the blood plasma'.

In 1963, Di Bella began his study of the relationship between blood platelets and the habenulae (nerve fibres connecting to the thalamus in the brain). The idea of exploring this area of research occurred to him while helplessly observing his friend's child terminally ill with leukaemia. 'Only someone like me would imagine – at that tragic moment – that the disease was somehow affecting the central nervous system,' he now admits. The idea of investigating this chemical relationship seemed illogical, and there was no certainty that it would produce any tangible results. Despite the many difficulties involved and the inadequacies of the hospital equipment, Di Bella nevertheless persisted in this research, with the help of his assistant, Deda. He managed to find, in the hospital, and repair, an old, broken Horsley–Clark stereotaxy machine, which allowed him to view the patient's brain in 3–D, and greatly assisted his research.

Di Bella has pioneered the use of melatonin in tumour therapy. In 1970 he was the first scientist in the world to recognise its potential in cancer treatment, when he suggested combining melatonin with somatostatin, retinoids and tocopherols (vitamin E).

In 1978, in Amsterdam, he publicised the results of his research, highlighting the inhibiting action on cell growth of melatonin, somatostatin and also bromo-criptine. Russel J. Reiter, Professor of Neuro-endocrinology, Department of Cellular and Structural Biology, at the University of Texas' Health Science Center in San Antonio, attended the conference. He was one of the first to take notice of Di Bella's work in the realm of melatonin and its application to cancer treatment and later went on to become one of melatonin's major advocates. At the time, he wrote: 'Professor Di Bella PhD. has used melatonin on different types of tumours for many years…the therapy seems to have produced encouraging results. Unfortunately this work has been heavily criticised by the scientific community…This group (Di Bella and colleagues) have more experience in the use of melatonin than any other in the world.*

Reiter has been researching melatonin for thirty years, and is the author of a book entitled 'Melatonin: Your Body's Natural Wonder Drug', which includes a chapter called 'Reduce your risk of cancer and heart disease'. He claims that melatonin is a 'master hormone', stimulating the release of a wide variety of other hormones from the pituitary gland and boosting the immune system. Reiter and his colleague Hing-Sing Yu (Director of the Biorhythm Research Laboratory, Division of Mathematics, Computer Science and Statistics, at the University of Texas) confirmed that, with regard to Di Bella's research, '...in all cases, melatonin was quite effective in causing substantial tumour regression or eradicating the disease altogether. Likewise, Di Bella and colleagues reported the successful use of melatonin in the treatment of patients with osteogenic sarcoma [malignant tumour of connective tissue, that forms new bone], lymphoma [tumour arising from lymphoid tissue], or leukaemia, as in those with carcinomas [spreading malignant tumour of epithelial (surface/lining) tissue] of either the lung, stomach or breast...**

In his notes from another conference in 1979,

---

* 'The pineal gland', Russell J. Reiter, *Progress in Brain Research*, vol. 52, 1979.

** 'Melatonin in the treatment of cancer', Russell J. Reiter, Hing-Sing Yu, *Biosynthesis, Physiological Effects and Clinical Applications*, CRC Press.

Russell J. Reiter writes, 'According to Professors Di Bella, Rossi and Scalera, melatonin may have utility in the treatment of thrombocytopenia [reduction in blood platelets] and possibly other blood dyscrasias [disorders of blood development] as well. Apparently the beneficial effect of melatonin in these patients relates to its ability to promote platelet production by megakarocytes [their originating cells], a question which these individuals have experimentally tested. This group has given melatonin to several thousand patients during the last decade and has never noticed any untoward effects... In a personal interview I had with Professor Di Bella and his co-workers, he stated that the usual daily dose for those suffering from thrombocytopenia was 1–2 milligrams of melatonin orally, with the dose divided between morning and afternoon. According to these researchers the success rate in ameliorating the signs of thrombocytopenia was very high, i.e. well over 50%. Di Bella and colleagues claim that melatonin may have beneficial effects in patients suffering from various types of leukaemia. Specifically, they have used melatonin to treat individuals with chronic and acute lymphoblastic [relating to lymphoblasts, cells producing lympho-cytes] leukaemia and also thalessaemia [type of anaemia] patients. On occasion melatonin is apparently given in conjunction with more conven-tional therapeutic agents. Also, during my discussion with Professor Di Bella it became obvious that he had administered melatonin by many different routes. It seems apparent that this group has more experience in treating patients with melatonin than any other. It is important that the explicit details of these clinical trials be published so the value of this mode of therapy can be properly evaluated by haematologists throughout the world.'*

Di Bella's findings on the role of melatonin were soon confirmed in successive meetings, in Brema and then in Athens in 1980. 'Di Bella used melatonin for the first time on a human patient in a case of haematological neoplasia (acute lymphoblastic leukaemia), a form of blood cancer. In the years following this first, successful application, it was used by others, in association with somatostatin and anti-oxidants, to treat other haemopathies (blood disorders) as well as solid tumours.'**

According to Di Bella, melatonin's biological properties are as significant as its therapeutic applications. Melatonin seems to be responsible for ensuring that certain basic functions are carried out and modulated at a cellular level. Melatonin is necessary in regulating bodily systems through the production of chemicals in the synapses (gaps) between individual single nerve cells. Via hydrogen bonding, billions of

---

* 'The pineal', Russell J. Reiter, *Annual Research Reviews*, Eden Press, vol. 6, 1981.

** 'The use of melatonin in neoplastic pathology', M. Maderena, S. Ciarletti, F. Goffredo, *Melatonin – From Research to Application*, papers from the conference, Reggio, Calabria, 25 January 1997

platelets nourish the cells of the epithelium (surface or lining tissue) through their indirect release and uptake of melatonin and serotonin. In Di Bella's opinion, melatonin is the most active of the platelets' natural anti-aggregants (which prevent clumping); he considers it a specifically targeted guarantor which maintains the normal properties of the blood and the trophism (nourishment) of the blood vessels (essential for a healthy circulatory system). It is unique in its ability to regulate exchanges between the blood and its surrounding tissues, ensuring an optimal blood composition and inhibiting the release and replication of growth factors and their receptors.

In short, melatonin can facilitate the curing of cancer. Although it is not responsible for cancer recovery in itself, and does not modify the nature of the cancerous tumour (its aggressiveness, its tendency to spread, the vital functions of the organs it attacks), 'Without melatonin,' Di Bella asserts, 'there can be no cure'. It is essential to the effectiveness of the MDB therapy.

Melatonin is able to permeate the molecules of the body within twelve days of being introduced into the bloodstream but, for it to be adequately absorbed, it must be taken in conjunction with the amino acid adenine riboside. The combination with this amino acid leads to the formation of hydrogen bonds which make the melatonin soluble and therefore promote its absorption. The preparation of soluble melatonin requires special equipment costing about £25,000. Using melatonin without adenine riboside can seriously jeopardise the efficacy of MDB. That does not mean, however, that dishonest pharmacies have not tried to sell poorly prepared melatonin to the unsuspecting patient.

Cancer is big business.

Somatostatin

Somatostatin is a polypeptide (protein with a particular amino acid formation) found in the brain (hypothalamus), pancreas (D-cells in the islets of Langerhans), stomach (mucosal D-cells), and small and large intestines. Although produced principally in the anterior (front) area of the hypothalamus, it may also be produced in other parts of the brain (cortex, encephalic trunk), spinal bone marrow, pancreas, some parts of the gastrointestinal tract, kidney and bladder. When it was first isolated in the brain it was thought to be only a growth factor inhibitor, but successive studies have shown that it possesses other, more complex functions, both endocrine and not.

The role of somatostatin is effectively to block the action of growth hormone (somatotrophin), produced in the pituitary gland. So important is growth hormone to growth, that, in many cases of dwarfism, the pituitary gland, and thus this hormone are found to be missing. Growth hormone anomalies are likely to be responsible for many cases of cancer.

In Di Bella's treatment, somatostatin's growth-inhibiting action is directed towards secretion of growth hormone in the pituitary gland. This slows down cancer cell growth while leaving healthy cells untouched. Di Bella claims that, with only 3 milligrams of somatostatin daily, he can successfully inhibit the activity of the growth hormone producing cells in the pituitary gland. The effectiveness of the treatment can be increased by varying the duration and the time of day of administration. Somatostatin is best given during the night, since at this time the 'bursts' of hormonal activity in the pituitary gland are more frequent and productive than during the day. Unlike other drugs, where the effect is usually heightened in proportion to the increased dose, this does not appear true with somatostatin – 3 milligrams seems to be the optimum dose to block the growth of the tumour, provided that the somatostatin is taken together with the other substances prescribed in MDB. Administered in this quantity it has no perceivable side effects.

Children must be given a smaller dose – in fact, the usual dose in their case starts at 0.25 milligrams daily and is gradually increased to 0.5 or 0.75 milligrams. The danger in that the somatostatin will interfere with the growth of the child and could possibly cause dwarfism. Di Bella believes that this risk can be largely avoided since tumours tend to appear only during a certain phase in childhood, and the treatment lasts only for a brief length of time. Continuing somatostatin treatment indefinitely in children is inadvisable, however, since it does cause temporary cessation of growth during administration. In such cases the therapy is prescribed for a limited period, thus initiating a process which will continue independently in the affected tissues and cause the tumour to disappear. Although the risk exists, Di Bella is not aware of any case of dwarfism being reported during the twenty or so years in which he has been using MDB successfully to treat children.

In order to compensate for the problem of the very brief half-life (duration of activity) of somatostatin, synthetic compounds have been produced containing additional substances which are able to prolong the period during which the drug is active in the body. In order to overcome that very same problem, Di Bella prescribes the administration of somatostatin using special 'slow-release' syringes, which allow the substance to be gradually absorbed into the body at a constant rate over a relatively long period of about 8 hours.

Somatostatin receptors are present in many human cancers, although there are high numbers of them in gastrointestinal tumours. Di Bella maintains, however, that the drug's action is not the same in all types of cells and systems and that these receptors represent only one way (albeit the easiest) through which the drug can be absorbed and take effect on cell growth. The professor therefore uses somatostatin to cure all types of tumours, with particularly encouraging results in those affecting the upper intestine, the duodenum, the liver and the pancreas.

During the Athens Conference in 1981, Di Bella described his research: 'We are using somatostatin, together with bromocriptine, melatonin and cyclophosphamide, in tumours of the breast, lungs, stomach, intestine, Hodgkin's disease, non-Hodgkin's lymphoma, malignant histiocytes [connective tissue cells], osteogenic sarcomas, neuroblastomas [sarcomas of the nervous system], and melanomas [skin tumours]... No side effects have been recorded after many years of treatment...we have numerous case studies to support the assertion that in many cases of metastasis [spreading] of cerebral tumours and breast cancers, a complete recovery has been effected. These excellent results allow patients to resume their normal lives with a significantly increased life expectancy... The cancer treatment based on somatostatin, melatonin, prolactin inhibitors [i.e. bromocriptine] and ACTH is probably the most naturally active of the treatments officially developed and applied. There is no apparent evidence of toxicity and the treatment is well tolerated.'*

Numerous articles and papers have been published in recent years by other scientists working independently of Di Bella's group, attributing significant anticancer properties to somatostatin. The following was published in 1996 in the American journal *Metabolism*:

'The potential role of somatostatin (SRIF) in the

---

* 'Somatostatin in cancer therapy', paper from the Athens Conference, 1–3 June 1981.

diagnosis and treatment of non-endocrine human cancers is being reviewed. There have been many reports of the growth-inhibitory activity of SRIF on normal and transformed cells in vitro [in the laboratory]. Many processes involved in malignant tumour growth depend on autocrine growth mechanisms and somatostatin receptors (ssts) are present on many human cancers. It is possible that mutations in ssts result in a loss of check on proliferation in cancer cells. SRIF analogs may have a number of roles in clinical oncology. Use of radio-labelled tracers enables imaging of tumours bearing ssts; newer agents may enable positron emission tomography (PET) analyses or may be used to deliver lethal radiation doses to cells bearing a unique subset of ssts. Although the ability of SRIF and its analogs to inhibit cellular proliferation has been shown in vitro, it has yet to be demonstrated in humans with cancer. Clinical improvements seen with SRIF or its analogs in cancer patients may be related to indirect effects on local production of growth factors and inhibition of tumoural angiogenesis [growth of blood vessels into the tumour]. Thus with regard to their potential therapeutic role, SRIF analogs are likely to be used only in conjunction with other approaches, such as radiation, immunotherapy, chemotherapy and growth-factor modulation. Further research into the fundamental functions of ssts and the intracellular actions of SRIF analogs will be needed to assess the potential usefulness of the latter in slowing the progression of human cancers.'*

This article refers to the commonly held belief that somatostatin can be effective only in the treatment of relatively rare endocrine tumours. However, it continues to underline the role of somatostatin in the diagnosis and treatment of other types of human cancer, and describes the conditions for its possible applications in oncology. As somatostatin receptors exist in many types of cancer cells it is therefore possible for the substance to intervene in the regulation of growth in a much wider range of cases than was previously thought possible.

Furthermore, the article highlights the fact that, for somatostatin to be effective in cancer therapy, it must be used in conjunction with other substances which promote its active properties. In Di Bella's treatment, this role is performed by melatonin and antioxidants, which are always prescribed with somatostatin, on the basis of their ability to regulate growth hormone.

Retinoids and vitamin A

Retinoids are deriviTives of vitamin A, a substance vital for growth and sight. They include both naturally occurring and synthetic forms. Retinoids have

---

* 'Somatostatin and Cancer', R. J. Robins, *Metabolism*, vol. 13
  (8), August 1996.

antiproliferative effects (discouraging cell multiplication) and may induce cellular differentiation. They are also used to treat specific forms of cancer.

Vitamin A is found in margarines, oily fish, liver and dairy fats. It can be synthesised by the body from dietary carotene found in carrots and green leafy vegetables.

The body requires vitamin A, sometimes referred to as the 'skin and membrane vitamin' and the 'growth vitamin', to guarantee the normal functioning of the epithelia, bones, reproductive system and for embryonic growth. It also has considerable growth-regulating properties. A deficiency in this vitamin, crucial for the skin and membranes that protect the body from all external and potentially damaging substances, could be extremely dangerous. Given the multiplicity of its actions and its pivotal role in the biochemistry which governs the body's functions, it is easy to see why vitamin A is fundamental to human life.

Since vitamin A regulates the proliferation of certain tissues, its anti-cancer properties have been studied for years. It has been shown that a lack of this vitamin in humans can increase the predisposition towards the formation of tumours.

Di Bella believes strongly in the importance of all vitamins. He claims that, among nutrients, perhaps the most important for growth and the control of it are the retinoids and vitamin A. He is eager to remind people that, even in ancient times, in Chinese medicine and in cures recorded around the time of

Hippocrates, 'powdered liver was used to treat various diseases of the ocular membranes and associated tissues, and we have since discovered it to be rich in these substances.

'Through its role in developing our sight, vitamin A affects circadian rhythms connected to perception of alternating light and dark. Through its genetic action it is instrumental in regulating cell growth and metabolism. It affects the base tissues of each of the three embryonic buds and has vital implications for the tissues protecting the skin and mucous membranes, not to mention various types of connective tissue.'

Di Bella notes that over a thousand types of retinoids have now been obtained synthetically. 'Their influence, which is effected through nuclear receptors, is capable of moderating the activity of our genes, and consequently cell differentiation and reproduction, even in cancers. Some of these derivatives (tri- or tetracyclines) have been proved to be a thousand times more powerful than retinol, the nearest natural equivalent.'

He predicts that the importance of similar compounds, such as citocalasine, will probably be recognised by science in the near future, and provide plausible explanations of mysterious anomalies in human growth patterns. 'It is not out of the question that, through the study of these similar substances, progress will also advance in cancer treatment. The application of particular retinoids has already put a good number of patients, facing the prospect of certain death, on the road to recovery.'

The composition of ingredients used in the MDB 'cocktail' is carefully calibrated to avoid the dangerous accumulation of any of the substances. The retinoid proportions used by Di Bella in his treatment are:

Retinoic acid (tretinoin):	1
Vitamin A palmitate (retinol):	1
Beta-carotene:	4
Vitamin E (alpha-tocopherol):	2,000

Retinoic acid and beta-carotene are used in their solid form while vitamin A palmitate (at room temperature) and vitamin E are used in their viscous liquid form.

The association between vitamin A and vitamin E is especially important as the presence of one increases the effectiveness of the other. Vitamin E (tocopherols) inhibits free radicals and has a strong antioxidant action in cells. vitamin E promotes the concentration of vitamin A in the liver and other cells. It has already been proved in laboratory tests on animals that vitamin E (found in vegetable oils) is able to block or slow down the formation of carcinogenic substances in the organism and affect the behaviour of tumours.

The following is from an article published in 1997 demonstrates that vitamin E, by determining the breakdown of cells, inhibits tumour growth through its selective action on the cells of the mammary glands and prostate:

'Recent reports have suggested that vitamin E may inhibit the growth of cancer and of the smooth muscle cells. We have studied the effect of dl-alpha-tocopherol (vitamin E) on a series of well-established cancer cell lines that included two erythroleukaemia [malignant disorder of white and red blood cells] cell lines and a hormone-responsive breast and prostate cancer cell line... Our studies thus give evidence of a general inhibition of cell proliferation by dl-alpha-tocopherol (vitamin E) with breast and prostate cancer cells distinctly more sensitive than erythroleukaemia cells.'*

Vitamin C (ascorbic acid) is a powerful antioxidant, and plays an important role in the stomach, where it inhibits nitrosamines, molecules which are potentially carcinogenic in high concentrations. Di Bella recommends taking generous doses in the form of supplements. It can be found in citrus fruits, potatoes and green leafy vegetables.

Vitamin D (cholecalciferol) is a fat-soluble vitamin fundamental in the treatment of tumours which attack bone tissue. It can be found in oily fish, margarine and some fortified milk.

Di Bella recommends avoiding the use of metal spoons with vitamins (particularly in the case of vitamin C) taken orally, in order to prevent oxid-

---

* 'dl-alpha tocopherol induces apoptosis in erythroleukaemia, prostate, and breast cancer cells', G. Sigounas, A. Anagnostou, M. Steiner, Nutr. Cancer, vol. 28(1), 1997.

isation. For similar reasons, he advises dissolving vitamin C in mineral water and not tap water, which often contains high levels of chlorine, destructive of many of the vitamin's properties.

Bromocriptine

Bromocriptine is a semi-synthetic ergot alkaloid from the group of lysergic acid derivatives which inhibit the production of the hormone prolactin, secreted from the pituitary gland. Bromocriptine has many hormone-like properties, although, from a bio-chemical and physiological point of view, it cannot be considered a hormone.

Bromocriptine, which basically restores the chemical balance necessary for normal nerve impulses, has a wide range of functions, and is widely known to retard tumour growth. Hence, it is used by many oncologists in the treatment of hyperpro-lactinaemia (increased prolactin in the blood) associated with various pituitary tumours. Other common uses of bromocriptine are in the treatment of Parkinson's disease, infertility, acromegaly (excess production of growth hormone) and premenstrual symptoms.

Prolactin triggers the production of milk in women after childbirth and is related to growth factors. In the treatment of certain endocrine tumours, such as those of the breasts, Di Bella advocates regular checks of prolactin levels in the blood of patients of all ages. He claims that prolactin levels in the blood can serve as an accurate indicator of the general health of the reproductive system, breast tissue and the potential appearance of breast lumps. 'Prolactin level checks performed on a regular basis,' he says, 'can be used not only diagnostically and curatively, but also prophylactically, particularly if they're begun in the first five years after the onset of menstruation. During that time various aspects of our hectic modern lifestyle can sometimes negatively influence the normal, healthy development of the breasts. A few tenths of a milligram of bromocriptine taken daily, together with a mixture of retinoids, can help to maintain the natural development pattern and check the growth of adenofibromas [type of tumour] which can occur at this point.'

The correlation between the anti-proliferative action of bromocriptine in NB2 lymphoma cells is one of the principles upon which the MDB therapy is based. In the last decade many promising new substances have started to be included in endocrine therapies for breast cancer, among them somatostatin and analogues of vitamins A and D, all of which have been used for years in MDB with overwhelmingly positive results.*

---

* 'Novel endocrine therapies in breast cancer', J. G. Klijn, B. Setjono-Ian, M. Bontenbal, Senaeve, J. Foekens, *Acta Oncol.*, vol. 35 (supp), 1996.

The extract reproduced below addresses the importance and effectiveness of prolactin-inhibiting drugs in the treatment of breast cancer:

'The growth regulatory effects of prolactin (PRL) on the human breast are mediated by its receptor (PRLr), a member of the cytokine receptor family... To confirm the role of this growth factor-receptor complex in normal and malignant breast tissues, the expression of PRL and PRLr was examined in parallel with the estrogen receptor (ER) and progesterone receptor (PR). Sixty-nine cases of primary invasive breast carcinoma were examined for PRL and PRLr expression by in situ hybridisation and immunohistochemical technique respectively. This data revealed widespread expression of PR and its receptor in the breast cancers studied and in the normal breast tissues, with no association between the expression of PRL-PRLr and ER or PR. These findings stand in contrast to prior radioimmunoassay-based studies that detected the PRLr in only 20-60% of breast carcinomas, most commonly in ER-PR-positive cells. These results confirm prior data indicating the presence of an autocrine/paracrine [types of endocrine] loop for the PRL-PRLr complex within the human breast. Pharmacological interventions aimed at the inhibition of function of this growth regulatory receptor complex may be of considerable utility in the therapy of this disease.'*

---

* 'Expression of prolactin and its receptor in human breast carcinoma' C. Reynolds et al., *Endocrinology*, vol. 138 (12), 1997.

Other scientists besides Di Bella have demonstrated prolactin's influence on many forms of cancer. A study (from the University of Brescia, Italy) was presented in 1995, stating that tumour treatment with bromo- criptine produced a 'normalisation of plasma prolactin and tumour regression'.*

Bromocriptine is administered orally and absorbed by the body within two to three weeks. It has been studied in cancer research both alone and with nerve growth factor. The drug has been used for treating pituitary tumours for 10–12 years without serious long- or short-term side effects. The majority of bromocriptine's adverse reactions (the most common being nausea) are dose related.

Other studies have resulted in similar conclusions: that bromocriptine is likely to play a significant role in cancer treatment. It just may provide the missing piece in the confusing cancer research puzzle.

---

* 'Nerve growth factor and bromocriptine: a sequential therapy for human bromocriptine resistant prolactinomas', C. Missale, M. Losa, F. Boroni, M. Giovanelli, A. Balsari, F. Spani. Department of Biomedical Sciences and Biotechnology, School of Medicine, University of Brescia, Italy, 1995.

A Step Forward

Di Bella's cancer treatment is the result of over three decades of his painstaking research, both theoretical and in the laboratory on animals and humans.

The anti-cancer properties of the four substances that make up Di Bella's 'tetralogy' are all currently being tested by other researchers, with promising results. Between 1995 and 1997 over 180 articles have been cited on Medline (computer database of medical papers) just regarding the role of somatostatin in treating cancer. Much of today's innovative work on cancer treatment includes one or more substances from the MDB. Furthermore, many other studies have stressed the importance in future cancer research of using a combined therapy.

Di Bella's therapy has no significant, unpleasant side effects, provided the drugs which make up the treatment are prepared according to the strict procedures the professor recommends. 'From my experience, and as far as I know, no-one has ever died as a direct result of this treatment,' he says. 'It is more affordable and less painful than chemotherapy or radiotherapy. Its administration requires no special equipment apart from a "slow-uptake" syringe.'

In MDB, the professor asserts that there are none of the frightening declines in leucocyte levels in the blood, or of haemoglobin in the red blood cells, which are seen with other therapies. Nor is there any noticeable and potentially dangerous decrease in the platelet count. The leucocyte counts of many of the patients who came to Di Bella after being treated with chemotherapy had reached levels as low as 500 (as compared to the 4,000 average needed for normal bodily functioning). He has been able to restore these patients' blood counts to normal in as few as 10-15 days of MDB.

Chemotherapy damages many elements fundamental to life, including the heart (an increase of up to 110-115 heartbeats per minute has been noted in patients after chemotherapy), blood circulation, and brain and kidney functioning. But Di Bella claims that his method is completely harmless to the body. 'Tests of the haemoglobin and hepatic [liver] functions during MDB also demonstrate its lack of toxicity,' he says.

Successful MDB treatment also promotes improvements in the metabolism of body tissues and in the functioning of the immune system. Positive, collateral effects of MDB are due to the other bio-chemical functions carried out by the treatment's principal components.

MDB substances administered by Di Bella have also provided significant results in a number of other illnesses, including epilepsy and Alzheimer's disease. Di Bella is convinced that a patient suffering from Alzheimer's disease can be treated effectively and resume a normal life, provided that the disease is caught early enough, and MDB treatment is begun as soon as the first symptoms appear. 'The condition,' he explains, 'can be treated with vitamin E in its purest form, with vitamin B1 and vitamin B12. An Alzheimer's patient can, under the right conditions, be successfully treated with these vitamins…I've seen magnetic resonance (MRI) scans which can confirm this. Doctors usually try to treat this disease with cortisone, but the results are misleading as they are often only temporary.'

Interestingly enough, the author's companion, a young woman called Carla, was diagnosed with epilepsy as an adolescent. After years of treatment involving unpleasant side effects, she discovered, after a thorough examination by the professor, that she was being treated with experimental drugs. Di Bella concluded not only that the medication she was taking seriously compromised her fertility, but that her problem was not, in fact, epilepsy. She was suffering from a brain lesion. She is currently following MDB alone, and scans show that the lesion has disappeared – and with it her convulsions.

Although MDB therapy has had an outstanding degree of success in the majority of the cases treated (both for cancer and other illnesses), Di Bella is careful to sound a note of caution. Not all cancers respond to the treatment and some respond better than others. Although the reasons are not yet understood, there are a few cases in which it has proved completely ineffective.

'Cancer,' he says, 'is the most complex expression of human cells and tissue formation, involving the highest functions of life. These functions do not depend on one single substance, but on a combination of substances and an immense number of reactions. Hence, the necessity of multiple substances to counteract these multiple reactions.'

A Hope for Humanity

Hope Starts Here

Via Marianini, where Professor Di Bella lives, is so tiny
that most visitors miss the turn-off and drive straight
into the centre of Modena. But those who find the
street instantly recognise the scientist's house (number
45) because of the crowds of people outside trying to
get in to speak to him. These men, women and
children come from all over Italy to meet the 86-year-
old creator of a treatment which has given hope to
cancer patients around the world. Many of them are
living in their cars and are prepared to die waiting
outside his house; others threaten to kill themselves if
they are refused treatment.

Luigi Di Bella has dedicated his entire life to
treating cancer. He spent the major part of his life
working seven days a week researching, seeing patients
and teaching. His time was, and still is, divided
between seeing patients and researching into cancer
and other intractable illnesses, in his laboratory.
Although he retired from his university teaching post

in 1984, Di Bella is still committed to helping the sick, who flock to him from everywhere.

The elderly Sicilian scientist was once able to treat all the patients who came to see him, many of whom had already been abandoned by their own doctors. He helped them as much as he could; and when he could not, because their bodies were too weakened by the effects of chemotherapy, he at least tried to give them more time and a little comfort. It has now become impossible for him to see the hundreds of patients that arrive at his door daily. He is forced to hang up a sign that he would have once considered unimaginable, announcing that he is no longer seeing patients. Only the people close to him understand how painful it is for Di Bella to refuse treatment to those who need his help.

The sick who come to Via Marianini have heard about the doctor through newspapers, television or word of mouth. Many are sent by their general practitioners or specialists, who have no alternative left to offer; others are referred by famous doctors and scientists who refuse to recognise him openly. The paients who arrive at his door are disillusioned by the empty promises of traditional cures – but they are not without hope.

The medical establishment, whose drug advisory council turned down five applications for Di Bella's method to be tested, is reluctant to sanction Di Bella's findings. Paradoxically, individuals in the medical community are starting to recognise the validity of the new road he is travelling, and appeal to him on behalf of their friends or loved ones.

A middle-aged man among the crowd in front of Di Bella's home displays a large sign expressing solidarity for the doctor. 'They killed my mother in twelve days,' he yells, approaching the house in the hope that the professor can see him, 'and then they locked me up in a mental institution because I asked why she died.' The people in the crowd turn the other way. They have their own problems.

The professor's house, which includes his laboratory, is modest but respectable, no different from the other houses on the block. Di Bella constructed the first floor himself in the 1950s. While building the house, he wrote letters to his wife in Sicily, telling her about the growing hostilities towards him in the university, and his need for a safe haven where he could work in peace and experiment with his new theories on cancer treatment. It was in this house that he began to develop his revolutionary cure. And he has slept in that same house every night since 1996, when he was attacked, presumably by those who stood to benefit by his removal, while returning to his apartment. Frequently, at night, he just stretches out in an armchair after hours of work.

Di Bella wakes up early every morning to do housework. At 7.00 a.m., he sees his first patient in his small office, which is filled from floor to ceiling with books and magazines, and decorated with photographs of Deda, his much-loved assistant who passed away some years ago. Now, the Professor almost never

leaves his house, except for his Sunday visits to the
cemetery, or for a medical hearing. With all the recent
publicity surrounding his 'cure', he can no longer even
walk in his little garden without being accosted by
journalists or prospective patients. One February
morning earlier this year, however, he decided to take
advantage of the cold weather which kept everyone
away, to take a turn outside with his daughter-in-law.
Two long-haired kids in leather jackets screeched past
on a motorcycle, as he came out, shouting, 'Go for it,
Doctor Gigi, you're great!'

Di Bella's patients, which now total over 20,000,
respect and adore him. Within the medical community, however, he is regarded with suspicion and
distrust. Talent often inspires jealousy, and the professor
is regarded as a brilliant and unique scientist. With its
significant financial interests to protect, the
establishment has done all it can to hinder his work
and tarnish his reputation. One celebrated doctor, for
example, reputedly called in all his patients who had
signed a pro-Di Bella petition, to personally repri-
mand them. Another physician who refused to
authorise a state subsidy for Di Bella's prescriptions
had a change of heart only when the weight of public
opinion and pressure from the media left him no
alternative.

Yet despite their outward show of hostility, doctors
and politicians tacitly acknowledge the professor's
expertise and continue to send their patients, family
and friends to him on the condition that their referrals

remain confidential. They publicly disapprove of him for refusing to disclose the results of his trials via 'appropriate' channels (which have already condemned his methods). But since the transmission of a television documentary in November 1997 and the massive public interest that resulted, the medical community in Italy and abroad has been forced to sit up and take notice of his thirty years of research.

The hundreds of letters that Rosy Bindi, the Italian Minister of Health, receives daily from patients and other interested parties demonstrate the support that Di Bella has gained. News of his dedication and altruism has reached all corners of the world, and he has been invited to live and research in Brazil, Canada, Argentina, Greece and many countries of Eastern Europe. The following excerpt is taken from a letter written by Maurena Lodi, whose mother was diagnosed with myeloma (cancer of the bone marrow) and treated by Di Bella:

August 8, 1997

Dear Minister of Health, Rosy Bindi,

For eighteen years, I knocked on the doors of specialists and hospitals around the world. I walked down dozens of corridors, and spent God knows how many days travelling, waiting for countless test results, examinations and treatments. The cynicism and insensitivity with which the most famous and respectable physicians treated my mother filled me with disgust and led me to profoundly question the integrity of the entire medical profession. I refuse to accept any sort of ethical judgement from that pulpit.

In 1978, my mother was diagnosed with myeloma. She was 46 years old. The verdict of the so-called medical community was unanimous: she had three years to live, at best. Some advocated chemotherapy, others recommended surgery. But the prognosis was still three, short years.

We consulted yet more specialists, and spent an unbelievable amount of money in the forlorn hope that, by listening to as many opinions as possible, our choice of treatment for my mother might somehow be made easier, or at least more educated. If only we had found one person who harboured even the tiniest grain of hope, it would have given my mother the strength to fight with dignity.

We met Professor Di Bella in 1979. At our first consultation, he told us in simple terms that myeloma was a slow, but relentless, disease. The best he could hope for was to decrease its growth rate which, given my mother's age, was rapid. He was extremely cautious, and made scrupulous checks, advising my mother to repeat even the most routine tests twice to ensure that the results were accurate. My mother was very ill, and the doctor entertained no illusions about her condition. He predicted there would be other unpleasant symptoms to come to terms with before she could hope to improve.

We followed Di Bella's cure for three years, despite increasing practical difficulties and the lack of support from the hospital staff. The illness stabilised, and my mother lived for another eighteen years, thanks to the doctor's professionalism and humanity. Di Bella never promised that the treatment would provide a miraculous recovery. He is neither a quack nor a profiteer, and has even refused to accept payment for his consultations. Nor is he a self-publicist, unlike some of his colleagues...

The Professor simply needs to be left in peace to continue his work with the support of the medical profession, and to be treated with the same respect given to other scientists.

Maurena Lodi

Recovery

Di Bella asserts that patients treated with MDB definitely improve, but that their degree of recovery depends on the type of cancer, and stage of its progress at the time of treatment. He claims to have an almost total recovery rate in patients with Hodgkin's disease. 'But,' he says, 'with tumours of the colon, rectum, pancreas and oesophagus, and those affecting the respiratory and digestive systems, we can also obtain positive results, as long as the treatment starts fairly early on. The same goes for melanoma.'

He stresses that some cancers can be large in volume yet be benign, while others can be small yet malignant and develop quickly. He claims that another variable in cancer treatment is the fact that cancer cells can also change with time. Therefore, in treating cancer and determining how responsive it will be to his treatment, he must study its individual behaviour, and its relationship with the secretory glands.

Most doctors, including Di Bella, agree that,

although we can inherit a predisposition to cancer, the major reasons why our bodies develop it are external: environmental or dietary.

The Importance of Diet

'The superficiality and inflexibility of the vast majority of advice given about diet is appalling. Much of what is said is not just ignorant but also unjustifiably prejudiced. Simple propaganda,' says Di Bella.

Having taught courses in nutrition at the university, the professor is particularly weary of the advice of 'popular dietology': 'Many of the diets published in newspapers and magazines contain recommendations which have no physiological validity whatsoever and are often lacking in elements which are essential for digestion, intestinal absorption and the digestive processes of secretion and incretion. It is a question of physiological ignorance, as usual, ignorance of the biochemistry of the intestinal tract and also of the elements of intermediate metabolism.'

Some of the suggestions that the professor makes (eating from the four food groups, avoiding fried and fatty foods, etc.) may seem like common sense, but he spends time emphasising and explaining them to each and every one of the patients he treats, just as he did with his students. It is, he reiterates, very important for those undergoing any cancer treatment to eat well so they can boost their immune system, cope with side effects, and fight infection. Only through good nutrition can the sick rebuild healthy tissue faster.

The professor also maintains that a sound knowledge of vitaminology is essential for all: doctors, specialists and patients. The in-depth study of vitamins and minerals requires scientific knowledge in a number of different fields. 'Everyone talks about vitamins, especially those who don't know anything about nutrition. Vitamins are basically chemical compounds, most of which are now produced synthetically in laboratories. They exist in both liquid and solid forms, and are absorbed by the body in the form of capsules or foods that contain them, through the intestine. Their name in fact derives from their fundamental role in the vital functions of the body.

'In cases of prolonged fasting or excessive consumption of certain foodstuffs to the detriment of others, the store of vitamins in the body can become depleted, leading to deficiency. Since vitamins function in quantities of milligrams or micrograms, the symptoms of deficiency appear slowly, gradually intensifying. Vitamin deficiency can eventually lead to death.

'Some animal species are able to produce vitamins in their own bodies, independent of their diet. Others, like guinea pigs, which are unable to synthesise vitamin C, develop symptoms of scurvy when fed a diet deficient in ascorbic acid [vitamin C] for long periods. Vitamin deficiency may be caused by poor supply of food, inadequate food consumption (slimming diets, anorexia), poor food absorption (intestinal disturbances, diarrhoea, removal of parts of the intestine) or excessive food consumption (which increases the metabolic rate).

'Each vitamin has a specific, characteristic function, as does its deficiency. A vitamin C deficiency, for example, causes weakening of the capillary walls and subsequently breakdown and haemorrhaging. Without an adequate amount of vitamin B, the functioning of the nerve cells can alter to the point of ceasing altogether.

'Diets where foods are overcooked, those lacking in fresh fruit and vegetables or those based on tinned, pasteurised and irradiated foodstuffs contain far fewer vitamins than those based on fresh foods, and can cause deficiencies over time.

'In practical terms, most vitamin deficiencies today are often multiple and simultaneous, and produce unusual, complicated symptoms which bewilder many doctors.'

Living with Cancer

Di Bella's method of curing illness revolves around putting the patient first and foremost.

His MDB is a complex system of physiological cure and patient care which has had overwhelming results in allowing the sick to live longer and in a healthier way. Di Bella believes that, under the right conditions, circumstances and with proper treatment, cancer is both curable and preventable. Although he believes strongly that his own cancer cure is definitive, the professer is willing to consider other 'alternative' treatments, 'as long as they achieve good recovery results and improve the quality of the patient's everyday existence.' He seems to reflect the open-mindedness of a great many others weary of the limits of modern medicine. A national telephone survey published in the *New England Journal of Medicine* in 1993 found that one in three Americans used unconventional therapies; the survey also found that Americans spent $13.7 billion in 1991 on alternative treatments.

To prevent cancer proving lethal, Di Bella insists that it is vital to intervene properly and as soon as the first signs of the tumour appear. 'To obtain the best results, treatment must be started as soon as possible and not after endless attempts to cure a tumour by other (often toxic) means.' With immediate and proper treatment, the professor claims that the cancer can be totally eliminated. 'I've seen a carcinoma of the pancreas disappear completely with my treatment. This is a very serious type of tumour because, if it begins to reproduce in this organ, it can easily release metastases into the lymph nodes, affecting the liver. And then things get very complicated. To date, this patient has not relapsed. However, similar cases, but where the treatment is not applied early enough, may not provide the same results.' He says that the medical practitioner really has an enormous responsibility in such cases, where the timing of the treatment, as well as the method itself, can be a matter of not just reducing suffering but of life or death.

Di Bella asserts that everything inside our bodies has to pass through either the skin or the mucous membranes which line the digestive, the respiratory, and the genito-urinary systems. 'Protecting our skin and other membranes from damaging toxins is already a great step towards effective prevention, but this action needs to be continued throughout our lives, not just for a day.' In his opinion, there is no better way of preventing disease than by an orderly, moderate lifestyle that does not exceed certain limits. 'If we were able to understand completely the nourishment and growth of the skin and membranes, then we would have a more concrete concept of cancer prevention. Otherwise, it looks like tumours will always be with us because, in a sense, we form them ourselves. We will probably never achieve prophylaxis that is 100% effective.'

Perhaps the most controversial side of the cure Di Bella has developed is his assertion that it is possible for patients affected with cancer to live normal lives even when their tumours have not completely disappeared. The professor claims to be treating dozens of patients whose tumour growth has been successfully blocked by the administration of MDB and who are now able to lead normal lives at home and at work despite the fact that the disease is still present in their bodies.

Di Bella suggests viewing cancer in the same light as any other chronic illness, such as diabetes or even schizophrenia. The important factor is to bring the tumour under control through the administration of the combination of drugs prescribed in MDB. 'This is a concept which is still being developed and one which will not be fully explored in my lifetime,' the professor says. 'Unfortunately, we have become tied to a tradition of trying to remove the affected parts completely; that is not always necessarily the best solution.'

A female patient Di Bella treated had a large, but perfectly encapsulated (enclosed) carcinoma in her right adrenal gland. Her previous doctor had operated on it, and the medical staff were all sure that the operation would be successful because of the nature of the tumour. After only three months, the woman's lungs contained seven or eight metastases. 'Under the circumstances it was a miracle her lungs were working at all.' After three years of MDB, the metastases were reduced to one half of their previous size. Years have passed, and she now leads a normal life. The woman has learned to live with her cancer. 'She looks at her x-rays, and is completely aware of her condition. There is not much to talk about when she comes to see me for her check-ups, two or three times a year. She has had neither a cold nor 'flu in the entire period of her treatment because MDB also protects the organism against viral infections."

Di Bella knows of many other cases of patients co-existing with their cancer. 'In breast cancer, for instance, I have treated many cases where women have preferred to keep their breast intact and accept their tumour (provided that it is contained and has not spread anywhere else), rather than face surgery. A mastectomy is a formidable psychological step for a woman to take. The breast is, after all, an important element of a woman's femininity. And the scars from radical mastectomies are often ugly and deforming, especially when the armpit cavity has to be emptied in addition to the main surgery. 'I try to help my patients choose the best possible treatment,' he says, 'preferably one which is compatible with their beliefs and emotions.'

In these cases, Di Bella asserts that MDB can produce excellent results. He admits, however, that, 'to some doctors, all this may seem far-fetched and incomprehensible. They have no patience with these sorts of sentiments. I don't pretend that with this method we can be 100% sure that the cancer will stabilise and the person's health will sort itself out. These cases are not as straightforward as if the cancer had suddenly disappeared altogether. However, if diagnosis is pronounced early enough and MDB therapy begun immediately, without recourse to other damaging treatments in the meantime, the results can be not only encouraging but really outstanding. In a relatively short time, the growth of the cancer can be blocked without any reason for me to believe it will develop further.'

Having successfully treated many cases similar to the above, Di Bella strongly believes that it is possible for the patient to live with cancer, with minimal danger of metastasis, for long periods of time. 'I remember a young man who came to see me. He was just 32 years old. His left leg had been amputated because of a sarcoma. He was just a boy, so young... After the amputation was performed the diagnosis stated that the cancer was already in metastasis. With the standard treatment, he was then ordered to go through chemotherapy as well. Either that, or they would have simply given up on him since the tumour in his lung which had developed by then was inoperable. I believe that that terrible amputation was unnecessary. They should have avoided it, and instead tried to find an alternative method of treatment which enabled him to live with his illness. The quality of that boy's life could have been so much better.'

Di Bella often cites the case of a patient he treated who was suffering from Grawitz's tumour (hyper-nephroma, kidney tumour). 'The tumour was spherical in shape and almost 20 centimetres in diameter,' he relates. 'It was completely encapsulated. The surgeon therefore thought that removing it would be a straightforward operation. No more than three months after the operation the patient's lungs were full of metastases. There was no possibility of operating again at that point, since the cancer was so widespread in the lung tissue that it would have meant practically removing the lungs in their entirety. There was nothing that so-called traditional medicine could do for her when I began treating her with MDB. That was four years ago and that lady is still alive today. She called me a few days ago to consult me about her condition. Do you know what she wanted to know? Whether it would be alright for her to go back to work.

'Another patient with cancer in both his kidneys came to see me. His case was very serious and, fearing the worst, I referred him to various oncology centres in Milan, Turin and Aviano. They all pronounced the same the verdict – they could do nothing for him. He was only 42 and the father of a young family. In desperation, he came back to me, and I prescribed

MDB, but without, I must admit, much conviction that he would recover. I explained his condition to him, and told him how I viewed his chances with my treatment. Now, eleven months later, the state of his kidneys is already substantially improved, and he is learning to live with his illness. The therapy he is following is compatible with a normal lifestyle, and he can stay at home without endless periods of hospitalisation.'

In cerebral (brain) tumours, particularly astrocytoma, Di Bella claims that the results which can be achieved with MDB are good, as long as the intervention starts at the appropriate point in the pathology of the disease and before the symptoms are too well established. 'Many of these tumours are inoperable due to their position, especially those situated deep in the bulbi. But I've been successfully treating patients with astrocytoma for many years.' He has also treated patients with tumours in other parts of the brain: the frontal lobes, the occiput and at the head of the caudate nucleus.

'I think we need to ask ourselves seriously whether or not it is accurate to consider cancer an inescapable death sentence? Are we really so powerless and ignorant that we can do nothing to intervene?' In his opinion, this negative attitude is unjustified. 'Why are we still making the same mistakes we've been making for decades, using radiotherapy, chemotherapy and surgery, which we know are often ineffective and damaging?'

Healing Stories

'Whatsoever house I enter, there will I go for the benefit of the sick, refraining from all wrongdoing... Whatsoever things I see or hear in my attendance on the sick which ought not to be voiced abroad, I will keep silence thereon.'

The Hippocratic Oath

Hippocrates, the most celebrated physician in Greek antiquity, took an oath before Apollo and all the other gods and goddesses; he swore to respect his father who had taught him all he knew, he promised to give his patients his light and his knowledge, protect them against all things which were harmful or unjust, and he pledged his complete discretion, both in and out of the realm of medicine.

The Hippocratic Oath embodies the duties and obligations of physicians and is usually taken upon entering the practice of medicine. It may now seem a mere formality to many medical graduates who pledge it — a collection of outdated rules of little relevance in a modern era of advanced technology, where medicine has assumed a distant, strictly scientific character, and the doctor-patient relationship has been radically formalised. Yet, we can begin to understand the philosophy behind Hippocrates' vow if we stop to consider the truly unique nature of this relationship. It is one in which the patient is willing to reveal, with unconditional trust, the most intimate details of his or her personal life, in exchange for the physician's advice and comfort. The relationship is based on mutual understanding and agreement and reciprocal obligations.

With the social evolution which has characterised the 20th century, however, doctors are often obliged to practise their profession in such unfavourable circumstances that the spirit of the Hippocratic Oath and the relationship it regulates have become so devalued that they seem divorced from reality.

The bombardment of pharmaceutical propaganda has prevented many doctors from providing patients with the best possible advice and treatment. At the same time, the average patient, whose doctor fails to provide a simplified explanation of medical terms, feels justified in criticising the medical profession. Both of these situations undermine the respected position of physicians in society. Paradoxically, however, many are still prepared to view doctors as omnipotent, and invest a quasi-religious faith in them. As a result, the uncured patient is often left feeling disoriented, abandoned and angry.

Young doctors today receive rudimentary training in developing and nurturing the doctor-patient relationship; they are forced to 'learn on the job' where self-instruction is inappropriate. In initial contact with patients, they tend to ignore case history details (the importance of which schools fail to emphasise) and rarely carry out rudimentary analyses. Consequently, the modern doctor focuses immediately on the symptoms of the illness – the fever, the pain, the cough – without giving adequate attention to the patient's overall state of health and medical history. University training emphasises the direct relationship between symptoms and medication; thus prescriptions are routinely authorised without further clinical or pharmacokinetic investigation. If the symptoms fail to respond and persist without noticeable improvement, the patient is then bundled up and delivered into the hands of hospital specialists, the radiologist or biochemist, for example.

The average doctor, victim of a complex, hectic and stressful daily schedule, is dissuaded from devoting excess time and energy to issuing a complete and thorough diagnosis for each individual patient. In sensing this, the patient may subconsciously refuse to accept his or her responsibility in the 'mutual contract': telling the doctor only part of the problem, or only fractionally following the advice received. The trust pact is broken. The doctor, on his or her part, is well aware that by working against the infrastructure of the medical field (the hospital or Public Health System) he or she risks disciplinary action, reputation or patient loss. In most cases, therefore, the doctor makes compromises, taking care to stay within the boundaries of that system which essentially provides his or her livelihood.

As a result of this general professional cynicism, patients are 'dealt with' as quickly as possible; and where a diagnosis is unclear or symptoms persist, a multitude of frequently inappropriate examinations and analyses are ordered by hospital specialists. With no alternative but to accept the doctor's referrals, the patient hopes that these often expensive tests will eventually solve 'the problem'. Often, however, these endless, detailed investigations fail to take notice of the whole picture, apparent only in a global interpretation of the results. The diagnoses prove inconclusive, and the tests are continued. This vicious circle leads to an overall increase in the costs of research and Health Service operation.

By contrast, total dedication to patient examination and treatment can result in diagnosis and therapy comparable to 'masterpieces in the Art of Medicine'. And when the patient has no qualms in placing complete trust in his or her physician, the benefits of accurately followed treatment become apparent.

Unfortunately, the obstacles in installing a therapeutic relationship between doctors and patients are numerous. Intriguing scientific theories announced daily capture the public imagination. Established notions can apparently, from one day to the next, be overturned by the myriad new discoveries in pharmacology and surgical techniques. In truth, these sensational breakthroughs require careful study, balanced evaluation and considerable perception on the part of the medic, who must make an educated assessment of their real worth.

If doctors today are to transmit the benefits from this ever-increasing number of therapeutic advances to their patients, they must keep abreast of the progress being made in the new frontiers of medicine. This is the only way to re-establish the position of respect and trust accorded to the doctor in society, and create a return to the original Hippocratic code of ethics and a renaissance of the true Art of Medicine.

Luigi Di Bella
30 April 1998

The professor places a great deal of trust in the patient's own role in his or her healing process, a concept which relates to the ancient Hippocratic Oath. 'Recovery can only be facilitated when the person concerned is willing to follow all the advice given, not only that of a medical–pharmaceutical nature but also recommendations about diet and lifestyle. In practice, trying to regulate a person's whole life is impossible but no real prophylaxis can be achieved without the patient's participation.'

But patient participation also requires doctor participation in terms of time and attention. Statistics claim that in the UK there are 350 oncologists to treat 300,000 individuals diagnosed with cancer yearly; thus every oncologist is responsible for following an average of 1,000 patients. It is no wonder that they find it difficult to dedicate quality time on an individual basis. Professor Di Bella spends an average of three hours on his first examination of each new patient that he receives. He stresses that the patient should be taking care of his or herself, and instils in them a positive attitude and faith in their recovery.

Michele Cosentino is one of the few doctors in Italy who currently prescribes the MDB. At a certain point in his medical career he could no longer bear to see patients dying of cancer, and began searching for an alternative to the ineffective treatments he was forced to prescribe for them. He says that using MDB has re-ignited his enthusiasm for his job, which is now, first and foremost, about curing the sick.

Cosentino is devoted to Di Bella, whom he views as a professional leader as well as an accomplished scientist and physician. Each week, Consentino takes the plane from Sicily to Modena to discuss his cases and new research with the professor. He is a young doctor but, like the professor, he feels that his profession is a sacred responsibility, a position of great privilege, and his friendship with Di Bella has only served to strengthen his convictions. He is constantly bombarded by telephone calls from patients who know that they can call him at any time, day or night. He has learned from his mentor to be emotionally supportive, giving and available, even at the cost of his own privacy.

He is perfectly aware of the antagonism of the medical community towards his mentor. He feels that doctors have travelled so far along one road of cancer research that they have 'forgotten about the other routes which were visible at the crossroads, a while back'. If he sometimes speaks in metaphoric terms, it is because he is a reflective man, prepared to look for answers wherever they may be. 'Science,' he believes, 'is immensely powerful and contains a limitless potential to change our lives, but for those very reasons we must be extremely careful in selecting, refining and, if necessary, jettisoning what we take from it.' He believes that the current research trends in traditional cancer treatment must be reviewed.

'My own experience with conventional therapies has been so depressing that I would rather avoid these means altogether. It amazes me that no-one wants to admit that patients are dying at a rate of about 70% with chemotherapy and other invasive treatments. If not from the cancer, which continues to spread even more aggressively after treatment, then from chemo-therapy's side effects. Professor Di Bella is trying to develop a philosophy of treatment along with his method.'

The main reasons behind the critical reception of the MDB treatment relate to the fact that the substances used in Di Bella's 'cocktail' have not been adequately tested according to standard medical procedures. Nonetheless, a wealth of progressive scientific literature already exists on the elements included in the therapy Di Bella hypothesises. The professor's cancer cure has also been criticised for including drugs (i.e. somatostatin and melatonin) originally developed for other medical purposes.

The professor defends himself by saying, 'If our results (cured patients) are unacceptable to the medical profession because they have been obtained without following their imposed rigid standards and procedures of experimentation, then I would like to point out that many of the world's most important medical breakthroughs have been made similarly. As N.J. Wald said, "Many people think that before one starts testing something in clinical practice one must understand how it works. That is a misconception. Many of the most effective agents in medicine were actually found to work well in clinical practice before their mechanism of action was understood."'[*]

In line with his strict code of ethics, Di Bella refuses, and has always refused, to accept money for his consultation and treatment of the sick. He is known to get offended if patients ask about his consultation fee. His answer is always the same: that it is he who owes them, since he learns something new with every case

---

[*] 'Retinoids, differentiation and disease', N.J. Wald, *The Foundation Symposium*, 113, Pitman, 1985.

he treats. 'I have a great respect for my profession,' Di Bella confesses. 'All of us must live, and we need money for that. But I had my teaching salary, and now my university pension that I've earned by working over the years; it is enough for my needs. I find it revolting to ask for payment from a sick person who needs my help, since the patient has often suffered so much already. Especially when that person is afflicted with a tumour.' Di Bella believes a doctor represents the most privileged figure in our society because he or she knows the patients' most intimate secrets and characteristics. 'A doctor deals in nothing less than life or death – and we only die once. That means his or her responsibilities are the greatest of any profession. To reduce that privilege to the level of pounds, shillings and pence... no, I think that's wrong. My patients often write me letters and that's rewarding enough for me – I find them truly moving. I am enriched by that, not by money.' The emotional responses Di Bella receives from patients, ex-patients and hopeful future patients have been overwhelming. They are embracing the 'cure', which unsettles and disturbs the equilibrium of the international medical community.

For some time now, the professor's son, Adolfo Di Bella, has been putting together a selection of correspondence from the mountains of letters the doctor receives every day. Most of the letters come from patients, who write to thank him, express solidarity or, more often, plead desperately for his help. Through these letters, the Di Bella family has become familiar with the world of human suffering. Many of the pages contain the indescribable anguish of the terminally ill and their devastated families, a suffering too often aggravated by the physical pain and disfigurement of the treatments they are forced to endure. But, on the other side, there is also a touching note of faith in many of these sad testimonies, a very human refusal to give up hope, even in the face of tragedy. Adolfo pulls out an example from the pile before him, written by the grateful mother of one of his father's young patients:

Dear Prof. Di Bella,

This is the second Christmas that we have been able to spend with our darling G., thanks to your goodness. It has been such a happy holiday, given her continuing progress, which is becoming more and more apparent with each new day. We would also like to thank Dr B., who has been scrupulous in following your instructions and is most attentive to G. We really don't know how to express our thanks to you, dear professor — words are insufficient to express the joy we feel as parents, seeing the change in our daughter. We can only say again, thank you, thank you, Professor Di Bella, from the very bottom of our hearts, and from G. herself whose gratitude to you is endless.

With all best wishes for the New Year,
M.

Adolfo has witnessed many of these heart-rending cases first hand. In May 1996, a man from southern Italy brought his wife, suffering from Hodgkin's disease, to Modena to see Di Bella. She was very weak and moved with great difficulty. Her desperation showed in the deep furrows of her pale face. The disease had taken root some time ago and, after undergoing a series of futile treatments, she no longer had the strength to fight. Doctors in Milan and Paris had told the couple that she would not live to see the summer. The husband then related how they had travelled hundreds of miles to see a celebrated haematologist, who took one look at the wife's medical records and, in front of his patient, told her husband that he might as well take her home – she had less than two months to live. On the way out, his secretary reminded the couple that the bill for their consultation came to over £100, and they were encouraged to pay in cash.

Adolfo was shocked by the story, and tried to comfort the couple while they waited to see his father. The woman's husband privately confessed to him that all he wanted now was that his wife should suffer as little as possible – he could hope for nothing more. They met with the professor, who ordered her to take a mixture of vitimins and hormones especially formulated for her condition. In December of that same year, the couple called the Di Bellas to wish them a Merry Christmas, and to tell them that the wife was feeling much better after following the doctor's treatment. To the amazement of hospital doctors, the examinations revealed later that year that her illness had completely disappeared.

Perhaps the most moving case that the Adolfo Di Bella remembers is that of a little Swiss girl who was referred to his father with an advanced cerebral tumour. Oncology clinics all over the world had given up on her. By the time she saw the professor, her condition was severely weakened as a result of drugs and chemotherapy. The child's parents first noticed that something was amiss in the summer of 1996, when the girl developed a slight squint. Her paediatrician told them not to worry, but she soon began to drag one of her feet. An immature hip joint was diagnosed. Unconvinced, her parents took her to another specialist, who performed an ultrasound examination which revealed a huge cerebral tumour, 6 centimetres in circumference, which her parents were told was inoperable.

They decided to travel to the children's hospital in Zurich to consult with a Japanese specialist. He advised a surgical operation, saying that, although there was some risk of damage to the optical nerve, it was their only hope. The operation lasted nine hours, but the subsequent ultrasound revealed that some of the tumour was still present. The histology test showed that the tumour was of an extremely rare type (called 'pilocytic multicentric astrocytoma'). Only 20 other cases had ever been documented. Doctors told the family that the tumour would respond to neither chemotherapy nor radiotherapy. The prognosis was that it would not expand, but by December it was larger still.

The family decided to consult a specialist in Pittsburg, USA, who recommended chemotherapy, although there was, admittedly, little hope of its effectiveness. In January 1997, the girl entered the Duke Medical Center in Durham, North Carolina, where she was treated by an oncologist specialising in the rare type of tumour that was affecting her; he had treated six of the twenty recorded cases. Successive doses of cyclophosphamide were administered and the cycle of drugs was ordered to be continued again in Switzerland. In March, another ultrasound was performed and revealed that her condition was worsening. The family was advised to resume the chemotherapy. By this time, the child weighed less than 12 kilograms, and her body was covered in sores. Permanently restricted to the hospital, her quality of life was abysmal. Her parents were beside themselves with fear and grief.

A faint ray of hope came when, by chance, the girl's mother saw a television programme about Di Bella and his treatment. As soon as the programme ended, she tried to telephone him. After three solid hours of calling, her persistence was eventually rewarded when she heard his voice on the other end of the line. She explained her daughter's condition, and he agreed to examine her. An appointment was made there and then.

When her parents first brought her to Di Bella's

laboratory in April 1997, the girl was so weak that her father was forced to carry her in his arms. Her hair had fallen out, and she was barely able to lift her head to look at the doctor. She could not eat and hardly slept. She weighed just 11 kilograms. Adolfo, who was present during that visit, saw that the professor was so overcome with grief that he could hardly speak. But Di Bella was also angry, furious that a child could be reduced to this state by the medical profession. The professor examined her frail and wasted body for over three hours. Her mother cried inconsolably throughout the examination and he tried to reassure her: 'Don't cry. I know what you are feeling. I am a parent myself. Her condition is very serious, I have to admit, but don't give up. You must be strong for her.'

The parents later described how, while they were following Di Bella's treatment, cancer specialists continued to call them from America, trying to persuade them to abandon his method and revert to the chemotherapy. They said that the child would be dead within three months if they continued with Di Bella's advice. The girl's parents were torn apart by these conflicting recommendations but the charisma of the old Sicilian doctor, his genuine concern for their child and his attentiveness to what they had said about her condition inspired them with confidence. In the end, they decided to persevere with his treatment.

The girl began the MDB therapy on 21 April. 'When she came to see my father again on 28 June,' Adolfo says, smiling, 'my wife and I were astonished.

We couldn't take our eyes off her. Her parents told us that, after only three days of my father's cure, she had already begun to move her bowels normally; after a week, she regained her appetite. She was able to walk around the room holding her father's hand and did it several times to show us how much better she was feeling. The girl's mother could hardly hold back her tears of happiness. They sent us a Christmas card later that year thanking my father for giving them the most joyful Christmas they could have hoped for.'

This case, along with four others, created a furore in Switzerland. The physicians who examined the girl there were amazed at her recovery and, although they had previously told the girl's parents to avoid Di Bella, they now instructed them to continue following the cure to the letter. That little girl is now five and lives with her family in the Ticino canton of Switzerland, where dozens of patients are following the Di Bella treatment. One famous Swiss oncologist recently decided to approve the therapy for his own patients. Another doctor using the Di Bella therapy in Novaggio has over 90 patients currently in being treated.

Those who testify to Professor Di Bella's kindness and medical bravura are numerous. In 1960, the Ferrari family (no relation of Vigildo Ferrari) moved into the house next door to Di Bella's laboratory and they immediately struck up a neighbourly relation-ship. Alfio Ferrari remembers the doctor as a cordial but private man who has grown increasingly reserved in recent years.

Ferrari recalls Di Bella working in overalls in his little vegetable garden. The professor, keenly aware of the role of diet in the prevention of disease, insisted that his family eat a large amount of fresh vegetables. One day, he took the entire Ferrari family to a lecture on food and diet in Bologna and later, during dinner, explained his rules for a healthy, balanced diet. Above all, he told them, 'You must never eat too much – the important thing is always to leave the table before you're full!'

The Ferrari family occasionally called on the doctor for medical advice, sometimes for minor ailments, sometimes for more serious problems. In 1981, Alfio's wife was found to be suffering from a tumour. She was taken to the infirmary in Modena, where she was operated on by a famous surgeon, but it was not a success. After the operation another specialist examined her. 'He told us quite brutally that she had less than five months to live.' They decided to take her to see Di Bella. 'When we eventually took her to Professor Di Bella, he examined her exhaustively for over two hours, an unheard of amount of time in our experience with other doctors. He listened to her heart, pressed upon her liver, took her pulse and measured her blood pressure for a quarter of an a hour. He did not request that she undress since he believes that it is an often unnecessary practice, one which is embarrassing and humiliating for the patient. Afterwards, he explained my wife's condition to us clearly and precisely, and told us how he predicted the illness would develop.'

Professor Di Bella prescribed a cure of melatonin and vitamins, which had a positive effect on the patient almost immediately, within days. 'Whenever our family doctor prescribed something for her, we asked Professor Di Bella for his opinion. He would investigate the composition of the prescribed drugs, and then confirm whether or not they were compatible with my wife's state of health. He often discovered that one substance or another was not appropriate and could be substituted with something else. I'd then go back to our family doctor and ask that he change the prescription according to Professor Di Bella's recommendations.' Alfio's wife continued to live a full and happy life until 1992.

In the 1980s, Di Bella also helped Alfio's brother, Giorgio, who was undergoing dialysis for kidney trouble. At the time, Giorgio was suffering from serious anaemia, a common complication among dialysis patients, and he required frequent blood transfusions. One day, the professor suggested that he ask the hospital to start giving him erythropoetin. This substance, also known as Epo, is a hormone which acts on the bone marrow cells to stimulate the production of red blood cells. It began to be used officially in Italy and across most of Europe some years later. Thanks to Di Bella's suggestion, Giorgio's anaemia was soon brought under control.

Even if the Ferraris had not had first-hand experience of their neighbour's medical expertise, they would probably have intuited his skills by the steady stream of patients and students coming and going to and from the laboratory in Via Marianini. As Di Bella's fame grew, so did the ranks of his supporters and the number of patients prepared to profess publicly their belief in the man and his cure. The Ferraris, like most of Di Bella's friends and relatives, are baffled by the controversy surrounding this modest man: 'We believe Professor Di Bella is a truly outstanding doctor and scientist. In 1985, we tried to get him an interview on television in order to explain his therapy to the general public. But it was impossible; they said that there wasn't enough interest in the subject at the time.'

The professor's friends never imagined that over a decade later his picture would be plastered across the front pages of all the major papers and that he would become a sort of *cause célèbre* in the Italian media. Nor did they ever think that he would be the catalyst which almost brought the Italian Health Care System to its knees, and caused the public to fundamentally question the medical profession. This unassuming man had the courage to take on the giant pharmaceutical companies of the world, denouncing them on live television for allegedly obstructing his treatments and profiting from diseases like cancer. He has caused hunger strikes and mass demonstrations, with people chaining themselves to the Congress building, and he forced the Italian Health Minister to do a u-turn and order official trials of his cure. He has received delegations from Canada, South America, and Japan, and has been invited by governments from all over the world to discuss his research. And yet, he wants nothing more than to lock himself in his laboratory and study ways to alleviate the suffering of cancer patients.

Another vociferous defender of the professor is Gloria Melotti, an active member of the Maria Teresa Rossi Foundation in Modena, an organisation for Di Bella's patients. She first came into contact with the doctor when her mother was diagnosed with breast cancer, and given little hope of survival. Her nightmare began with harrowing, but ineffective, traditional cancer treatments. 'At the time, we didn't know about Professor Di Bella's therapy, and the medical staff who were aware of it merely advised us to keep up with the chemotherapy. In the same breath, they said that my mother was so far gone that it would be useless for me even to seek a second opinion.'

She and her mother were sitting in the hospital corridor when a patient who had been having chemotherapy was wheeled past. Her mother then confessed that she would rather die than be reduced to that state. Strangely enough, around that time, Alfio Ferrari telephoned Gloria on a work matter. In the course of their conversation, she mentioned her mother's illness, and he told her about his neighbour, Professor Di Bella. A few days later, they had their first appointment with the doctor. 'He examined my mother thoroughly, and the treatment he prescribed kept her alive for another four years. The quality of her life was much better than anything she could have expected on chemotherapy – she went dancing right up until the last weeks of her life.'

But their controversial decision to follow Di Bella's therapy was beset with problems. 'Our family doctor, who was also the President of the Medical Board in our province, not only advised my mother to be treated with chemotherapy, but he also refused, point blank, to sanction the somatostatin prescribed by Di Bella as the basis of his cure. The drug was still available in pharmacies then (now it is more difficult to find due to the high demand for it), but you needed your general practitioner's prescription to buy it at a government-subsidised price. 'We were willing to buy it at any price, though, because both my mother and I trusted Professor Di Bella completely.' Luckily, another doctor agreed to prescribe it for them, and so they were able to obtain it relatively cheaply. 'At the various hospitals and clinics where I took my mother for tests, doctors told us that Di Bella was nothing better than a witch-doctor and we'd soon be sorry that we'd been taken in by his fake treatment.'

Ivana B. is 43 years old and has had a successful career as a trade union representative. In the summer of 1996, she was diagnosed with the blood cancer myeloma, an excessive proliferation of antibody-producing plasma cells, which infiltrate the bone marrow. Ivana was terrified when her illness was first diagnosed. But she was absolutely certain of one thing – she was not going to let herself be treated by chemotherapy. 'I was more scared of the treatment than the disease itself. I didn't know what to do, my future seemed hopeless,' she confessed. 'And then I was lucky enough to hear about this amazing man, Dr. Di Bella, and suddenly my will to live returned – I was given hope.'

Ivana's illness has been under control since starting MDB. She spends about £200 a month on the drugs prescribed for her by Di Bella. The sum, miniscule compared to the cost of chemotherapy and radio-therapy, varies considerably depending on the dosage of somatostatin prescribed and its frequency. (Ivana has to take it only once a week.) She thinks that an important aspect of any treatment is also how the patient feels taking it – his or her quality of life and psychological state. 'I'm currently coming to terms with living with my disease, in line with Di Bella's philosophy,' Ivana says. 'Other experts would have said my cancer needs to be treated with surgery or systematically destroyed with chemotherapy. But if I can live for another thirty years like I'm living now, I'll be happy.'

Her experience has altered her perspective on patients' rights. 'It's horrible to hear all these doctors talk about cancer sufferers as if they're a bunch of simpletons who understand nothing about their illness and will believe the first thing any quack tells them. We don't think Di Bella is offering a free trip to Lourdes – we can weigh the possibilities of his cure for ourselves, and we should be allowed to make the choice of whether or not to try it. The sick should be allowed to have a say in how they want to be treated, whether in the public or the private sector. They should be fully informed about all their possibilities so that they can make an educated choice.'

The medical establishment's greatest fear is, in fact, that cancer patients will abandon conventional treatment in the hope for a 'miracle cure'. Most patients, however, are like Ivana. They have a clear idea of their needs, and are aware of the risks involved in any cancer treatment. They simply want the right to choose for themselves.

Ivana is reassured to know that 86-year-old Professor Di Bella has been taking melatonin himself without side effects, for almost forty years. 'I don't see why the government is so reluctant to make Di Bella's cure available for those who want it, at least. How long might national testing take? People with cancer do not have the luxury of waiting until the day it is officially sanctioned,' Ivana says, in tears. Her main worry at the moment is for the patients currently using MDB who are not judged 'eligible' to continue using it under the new (Italian) rules for official clinical trials (mainly conducted on the terminally ill). To have had their hope restored and then suddenly snatched away again is doubly cruel.

Emotional accounts of this kind have helped nurture an overriding feeling of support for alternative cancer cures and scepticism towards doctors, who often arrogantly impose their conventional treatments on sick, frightened and desperate patients. Di Bella, unlike those who may be perceived as cold and profit-motivated professionals, has dedicated his life and career to one purpose. 'It isn't a thirst for glory or the desire to make money that pushes me to devote myself to investigating new methods,' he says. 'It is the need to be able to offer some comfort to those who are desperate, those whose only prospect is a slow and inevitable death. It's the hope of being able to put an end to that disheartening professional impotence, poorly disguised by ambiguous claims and imaginary promises, that faces us all when we're confronted with this illness. In short, to put an end to human suffering.'

The Media Circus

When it was announced in early December 1997 that Professor Di Bella would be participating in a live TV talk show to clarify the issues involved in the 'Di Bella Affair', the Italian press talked of little else for days. The whole discussion surrounding MDB, the medical establishment's arrogant dismissal of the professor's work and the question of the 'right to choose' for cancer sufferers seeking treatment was the lead story in all the major dailies, and public interest was whipped to fever pitch.

Millions of Italians were glued to their television sets the night that the first interview with Di Bella was aired on national television. His uncompromising morality, and total disregard for personal gain, soon became apparent in the course of his debate with the five other professors brought in to defend the position of the medical establishment. The show struck a chord with the public's distrust of the Health Care System. For the professor, it was a personal but rather hollow victory: many people were still unclear as to what the therapy consisted of, which doctors would prescribe it, where the necessary drugs could be obtained and the contents of the 'sample clinical records' referred to during the programme. One thing was for sure, however – the public wanted to know more.

The morning after the transmission, Dr Silvio Garattini, Di Bella's major adversary (he declared the MDB to be 'a limp salad of words') and a member of the elite government advisory body, the Premier Health Council, flew to Rome to call an emergency council meeting. The encounter resulted in a memo to the Minister of Health, Rosy Bindi, recommending, firstly, that she suspend the market supply of the substances used in Di Bella's therapy and, secondly, that she avoid creating investigative committees relating to the MDB.

Throughout December the political side of things started heating up. On 23 December, Health Minister Bindi sent an ordinance to Di Bella requesting that one hundred clinical records of his be handed over immediately. He resisted in the name of patient privacy, so she threatened to send officials to his laboratory with a warrant. A few days later, in Florence, 35-year-old Eugenio Rivaira, an ex-patient of Di Bella's, volunteered his medical records to the authorities as a show of his solidarity with the doctor. He was the first of many.

Eugenio had visited Di Bella after successive cycles of chemotherapy left him weighing less than 40 kilograms. He had been ill since 1980, and his disease was, at that point, very advanced. Di Bella confirmed the hospital's diagnosis of malignant histiocytosis but said that, with MDB, Eugenio may still have a chance. After six days of scrupulously following the doctor's instructions, he had already gained 6 kilograms. A few months later, he was back at work. Today, eighteen years later, he is considered fully recovered.

Eugenio's decision started a chain reaction, and other patients soon came forward to volunteer their records. One of those was Otello Manzini from Modena, a sprightly 78-year-old. In his 1996 tax declaration, he claimed to have spent almost £4,000 on the drugs he needed to stay alive. Now, thankfully, his condition is much improved and he is managing on melatonin and a vitamin E compound. But in the past, his treatment had included somatostatin and he was forced to pay through the nose for it, as the state refused to subsidise the professor's prescriptions. 'I'm a pensioner,' he said indignantly. 'How can I afford to spend that sort of money? I tried in every way I could to get the drugs prescribed through the National Health System, but they wouldn't hear of it.' Despite his problems, Otello persevered with the Di Bella cure because he was convinced that it was a viable alternative to the surgery other experts had advised for the growing tumour in his vocal chords. 'I was treated with MDB and I survived. I haven't regretted it for a minute.' He cannot understand all the pandemonium surrounding Di Bella. 'He's a great scientist,' he says, 'and he deserves recognition for all the incredible work he's done to save people.'

While the lawyers debated the legality of the government's decision to temporarily suspend the supply of somatostatin to patients until the official trials were completed, outraged district health services in various parts of the country began to take matters into their own hands. In the southern region of Puglia, they decided to supply somatostatin free of charge to resident patients in their area, causing an uproar as desperate patients from all over the country flocked there to try to alter their residence status.

Marcello Baglioni experienced it all at first hand. Afflicted by a form of chronic leukaemia, he decided to abandon traditional cures some time ago. After numerous difficulties, he managed to obtain an appointment with Di Bella. The form of MDB therapy prescribed for his condition, after a lengthy examination, included substantial doses of somatostatin. Says Marcello, 'It became like the quest for the Holy Grail – I went the length and breadth of the country to get the stuff.' His own general practitioner agreed to write him a certificate indicating the advanced state of his illness, to take to his local hospital as proof that he genuinely required the drug. 'I arrived in the oncology department,' he says, 'and the consultant told me in no uncertain terms that he was not authorised to distribute somatostatin under the circumstances. My only alternative was to apply in the Piedmont region, where, he believed, they had taken a different stance.'

Some friends of Marcello's from Puglia then called him to tell him the news of their regional council's decision to make the drug available to its residents. He therefore decided to change his residency temporarily and brave the bewildering bureaucracy which this move entailed. He left for the South as soon as possible. By 31 January 1998, he had reached Brindisi and that Monday morning he entered the regional council building to file his request. His grim determination was rewarded on 5 February at 9.00 a.m. when, having badgered innumerable officials and filled out reams of forms, the pharmacy in Ostuni hospital gave him fifteen 3 milligram phials of somatostatin free of charge.

Marcello's story is the tip of the iceberg. The migration of patients and their families in search of this elusive substance has now become a mass phenomenon, along with the simultaneous emptying of hospital oncology departments all over Italy. Television appeals for calm, entreating patients not to leave their home towns, have fallen on deaf ears. Meanwhile, fewer and fewer experts are willing to be quoted publicly as advocating the effectiveness of chemotherapy and other traditional treatments.

Strangely enough, no-one has yet convincingly contested the effectiveness of somatostatin itself: the polemic is all related to the conditions restricting its availability. Oncologists are reluctant to air their opinions – pro or anti – even of the much-discussed melatonin. The subliminal messages generated by this behaviour are slowly filtering through to cancer sufferers, whose faith in the medical profession at large has reached an all-time low.

On 13 January 1998, a second televised debate with Di Bella as guest speaker was scheduled. This time, the Health Minister Rosy Bindi was also persuaded to participate in a face-to-face encounter with the professor. The programme represented yet another popular success for Di Bella, while an obvious sympathy sprang up between the professor and his 'adversary', Ms Bindi. In fact, the relationship of mutual respect established on the air was to continue via telephone and fax, with the two communicating almost every day during the endless debate on the official trials. Ms Bindi became, for Di Bella, 'the only one out of the lot of them with whom I can at least talk'.

During that month (January 1998), Di Bella made yet another demonstration of his altruism at the same time that the Minister of Health finally approved the official clinical trials of his treatment. The professor delivered the fruits of his life's work (the formula for his MDB treatment) along with all the documentation), to the state authorities. He could have earned millions of pounds had he patented the treatment – but he chose not to do so. The last time medical science witnessed such an unselfish act was in the 1960s when the American microbiologist, Albert Bruce Sabin, renounced the patent on his polio vaccine so that the entire world could receive it free of charge.

By mid-February, public hysteria was sky-high. Rumours abounded that the state statistics on cancer recovery had been manipulated and that, in reality, only one in two victims survived. Then the actual definition of 'recovery' in these figures was questioned, and whether even fewer patients receiving traditional therapies had survived. Mistrust of the medical structures, both public and private, involved in the fight against cancer was now growing out of all proportion.

The frenzy continued. Ansa (the Italian newswire service) issued a statement, which later proved to be erroneous, that a film starring Kathy Bates (as Rosy Bindi) was in the pipeline. There was talk of international experimentation, death threats and falsified documents. The professor suddenly found himself unwittingly manipulated by a series of consultants and hangers-on with their own interests in mind.

Despite official governmental cooperation, the national trials of the MDB leave much to be desired. An international committee was formed by the Italian Health Ministry to supervise them but, once the trials actually began, the members of the committee, which supposedly included Gordon McVie (Scientific Director of the London Cancer Research Campaign, and President of the European Organization for Research and Treatment of Cancer), were never again called upon. The methodology of the trials is questionable. It is even rumoured that there is no random patient selection, and no control group. It is also unclear whether or not one of the governmental protocol documents actually contains Di Bella's authentic signature.

The Italian parliament and Health Care System seem to have lost control of the 'Di Bella situation'. Many patients are falling into the greedy hands of charlatans and con artists who purport to be disciples of the professor, and use his name to make money out of the sick. A black market is flourishing in melatonin and in photocopies of prescriptions stolen from the doctor's patients. Racketeers are importing somato-statin into Italy from abroad, and selling it at astro-nomical prices.

Many feel the situation of public furore and discontent has been brought about by a mediocre Health Care System based on an inept, cumbersome bureaucracy and dictated to by the economic power of the pharmaceutical industry. But, while the infra-structure of the health services is crumbling, 160,000 people die of cancer annually. Since 1977, three million have died of various cancers. During all this time, Di Bella's treatment has existed in more or less the same form as he prescribes today. In 1973, the professor's detractors were able to suppress interna-tional publication of a report detailing his cure. If they had collaborated with him instead of side-lining his ideas, perhaps many thousands of cancer sufferers could have been saved.

The official statistics state that 50% of those afflicted by tumours now recover, thanks to 'new' therapeutic techniques based almost exclusively on chemotherapy, radiotherapy and surgery. But Di Bella dismisses these statistics by saying, 'They mean nothing – you get a much clearer picture from talking to people. Almost everyone has had direct experience with this disease, either in their own family or with someone they know well, but you'd be hard pressed to find more than a few long-term survivors. When we look more carefully at the figures, the truth emerges that, in fact, they only refer to those who have survived for up to five years. And there is no mention of the awful quality of life that many of those survivors are forced to endure. And what about those 'cured' of cancer who die of the side effects of chemotherapy? Is that what you would call effective treatment? If the TV cameras were suddenly given unlimited access to oncology and haematology wards, there would be a public outcry!' Apart from that, citizens continue to pay taxes which are supposed to help finance research into this disease – research which is turning up little.

Pharmacist Vigildo Ferrari feels that, 'The only progress made in the last thirty years is in surgical techniques, but they are applicable to only a minority of cases. According to recent parliamentary reports, the real recovery figures are more in the region of 4%. We can only hope that the Minister of Health will decide to open an investigation to throw some light on these numbers – we've been going ahead with these conventional treatments for half a century and they're just not providing us with positive results.'

The professor's youngest son, Adolfo, is convinced that much of the scandal which the Di Bella affair has ignited is due to the defensiveness of a limited number of influential specialists, defenders of traditional cancer treatments, who foresee their reputations and livelihoods crumbling and fear they will now be forced to concede to Di Bella. They may even have financial interests at stake. Many of them, handsomely rewarded by pharmaceutical companies for their collaboration, are afraid they will lose their prestigious positions if they are unable to keep drug industry interests to the fore.

But the weight of public opinion is swinging against them. Half of the Italian parliament is up in arms and the press is reluctant to support shady drug company tycoons and self-interested health officials. 'They can set up all the investigative boards, ethical committees and new organisations that they like to try to address the basic human rights which are at issue here, but the floodgates have already been thrown open,' says Adolfo Di Bella. 'It would be much more advisable to let alternative therapies like MDB co-exist with traditional ones, giving the educated patient the right to choose how he or she wants to be treated. In the meantime, people are dying out there and government is wasting time in useless argument like this, which is criminal.'

Professor Luigi Di Bella has been criticised for failing to publicise his research through the official scientific channels, an ironic accusation when he has been subjected to intimidation designed to prevent him from publishing his controversial studies (much of his work has had to appear in the guise of university theses or special papers). In order to make his studies available, he has been forced by celebrated hospital consultants and university professors – a number of whom owe their success to his assistance – to publish under their names.

In the light of the discoveries Di Bella has claimed to have made, surely one must ask whether such cast-iron conventions are not obstructing new thought and methods of research. As Albert Einstein himself remarked,' If you want to become a great scientist you must think for at least two hours every day in a manner completely opposite to that of your colleagues'.